Dr. Kaskel's
Living in Wellness

Volume One

Let Food Be Thy Medicine

Larry Kaskel, M.D. and
Michael Kaskel, R.N.

ISBN: 978-1-4834-0714-2 (sc)
ISBN: 978-1-4834-0713-5 (e)

Because of the dynamic nature of the Internet, any web addresses or links contained in this book may have changed since publication and may no longer be valid. The views expressed in this work are solely those of the author and do not necessarily reflect the views of Northwestern Medical or any of its affiliates. They also do not necessarily reflect the views of the publisher, and the publisher hereby disclaims any responsibility for them.

Any people depicted in stock imagery provided by Thinkstock are models, and such images are being used for illustrative purposes only. Certain stock imagery © Thinkstock.

Lulu Publishing Services rev. date: 04/29/2014

Dedication

We dedicate this book to our father, Albert Kaskel, who dedicated his life to teaching biology and writing science textbooks and in whose footsteps we humbly follow.

Contents

INTRODUCTION

"Let food be thy medicine and medicine be thy food" was wisdom first canonized by Hippocrates[1], the ancient Greek physician. It is advice that, to this day, has not lost its validity. *Let Food Be Thy Medicine* and the recommendations herein are inspired by my own observations and validated by the research and writings of many experts.

Eating according to the guidelines outlined in this book will not necessarily extend your life. If that happens, fine, but that isn't the thrust of this book. This book is meant to help you in making better choices about the food you eat so that you can improve your cellular health and help you cure yourself of chronic disease. In addition, changing how you eat by following the eating prescription outlined in these pages will make you feel better and improve your own quality of life.

Like most physicians writing about nutrition, I learned the medicinal value of food the slow way. Unfortunately, Hippocrates' wisdom is not an integral part of Western medical training. When I was in medical school 25 years ago, I had just just four hours of lectures on nutrition. While the tide is starting to turn, medical school training still lacks coursework on functional nutrition. This book is derived in part from a curriculum that I am developing for a medical school course on Lifestyle Medicine that I hope to teach in the future.

The book you're reading is *Volume One* of *Living in Wellness*. In it you will find information that we give our patients, you will read some of the blogs I've written over the past 5 years, you will read the transcript of an interview with a leading researcher in the field of cholesterol, and you'll be introduced to recipes created by a world-class, James Beard-inspired chef that are compatible with the types of foods you should eat. This is not a diet book. This is a book about the way you should eat for the rest of your life. There is no end until the fat lady sings. It is ongoing.

---

[1]   **Hippocrates,** (born *c.* 460 BC, island of Cos, Greece—died *c.* 375, Larissa, Thessaly), ancient physician who lived during Greece's Classical period and is traditionally regarded as the father of medicine.

Volume Two of *Living in Wellness* will deal with the mental and spiritual aspects of achieving wellness and is a future publication.

Larry Kaskel, M.D.
Chicago, 2013

ONE: How I Got Here

My path to understanding the importance of eating real food in order to attain and sustain good health was not straightforward. I, like most of my colleagues, routinely prescribed medications to treat the conditions of high blood pressure and high cholesterol. In fact, I considered myself an expert in treating high cholesterol and became board certified in lipidology—which is the study of cholesterol, fats and rare metabolic diseases.

Only after I started a lipid clinic did I begin to question the efficacy of the recommended conventional medical treatments for high cholesterol and high blood pressure. Even though in taking the medication many of my patients were able to arrive at the current target goals for blood pressure and cholesterol, I did not observe them experiencing better health. In fact, many of my patients that had successfully arrived at the target levels suffered fatigue, muscle aches, sleep apnea, erectile dysfunction, low energy and memory lapses.

To my surprise the more I treated patients with medications for these conditions, the more I observed their suffering with other issues. Many could not tolerate the numerous pills and medicines required to get them "to goal." Then, more puzzling, there were patients with cholesterol levels above the target numbers but who were in all other critical respects in good health and for whom I recommended cholesterol-lowering statins who then suffered complaints where they'd had none before. The medications created illness! Although not statistically relevant, these observations prompted me to investigate further.

Around that time I also began hosting a radio show on ReachMD XM called *Lipid Luminations*, where each week I would interview lipid experts on their recent studies or research.[2] The show gave me access to top expert physicians in the country. I studied hard before

---

[2] Here is the link for over 300 shows that I hosted during my tenure there:
http://www.reachmd.com/xmradioguest.aspx?pid=288
one of my favorite and most important show is included in the addendum.

the interviews and asked probing questions about the research my guests conducted. While some of the guests engaged with the questions I put to them and acknowledged the limitations of their respective studies, others became defensive, their arguments empty, their conclusions overstated, and their interests tainted by relationships with the pharmaceutical industry.

I learned how to deconstruct and analyze the statistical biases of scientific studies. Where the experts focused on something called *relative risk*, which is statistical jargon that, in this context, allows for the exaggeration in improvements from medication, I sought information about *absolute risk*. I wanted real numbers regarding the efficacy of statins, but not one of my expert guests could explain why patients continued to have heart attacks, strokes and die despite taking their miracle statin drugs. Something was amiss.

Then, in 2008 I attended a lecture by Mike Katke, cofounder of Metagenics, a nutraceutical (nutrition—rather than drug-related therapeutical) company, and had my *aha* moment. Katke had a food-based system founded upon the already known, well-proven, studied and recently reconfirmed Mediterranean Diet that actually worked.[3] It was just as Hippocrates had said, "Let food be thy medicine." I went back to my lipid clinic and immediately incorporated what I call the Lifestyle Program as an additional treatment.

My *aha* moment was followed by observation. The first patients that began the program significantly improved their metabolic health within the first 3 weeks. With very minimal fat loss, by following this program, they reversed their metabolic conditions. In fact, I was able to discontinue some of the medications they had been previously prescribed to control one or more of their chronic conditions. This is when I directed my focus towards using food as medicine.

---

[3] See this link to the most recent study done: http://www.nejm.org/doi/full/10.1056/NEJMoa1200303

TWO: The Lifestyle Program

With the help of my brother Mike, in our clinic *lifestyle medicine* became more than a tag line. I knew that for the program to succeed patients would have to be educated about the wisdom of eating good, healthful food. The initial 12 weeks of our program does exactly that. In that time, patients are taught how food can be their medicine and that they can effectively cure their chronic conditions by choosing foods that restore good metabolic health. Because many of the food choices we endorse in our program are in direct opposition to national guidelines and to those which are touted as healthy, the educational aspect was and still remains difficult. Our program, for example, recommends bacon and eggs for breakfast, and excludes even steel-cut oatmeal. Just as in the coaching of a ball player with a bad swing, we had to reeducate patients about the fundamentals of nutrition.

To do this the program we created incorporates weekly visits and ongoing support by lifestyle educators and other mid-level providers. Mike has been instrumental in hands-on teaching and guiding about proper nutrition. It is by virtue of his working side-by-side with me in the lifestyle intervention trenches, that I have been able to reach and help my patients. I credit Mike's partnering in this endeavor for my now having the time and the tools to provide true lifestyle medicine.

Here is how the program works in a nutshell: I see and examine patients, diagnose their condition, which can be prediabetes, diabetes, hypertension and/or obesity. I ask them if they want to manage their condition with medicine or if they would like to cure their condition and eliminate the need for at least 50% to 90% of their medications. If they opt for the latter, I prescribe the Lifestyle Program and introduce them to Mike or other educators to help them incorporate the program in their lifestyle.

It is remarkable what we have been able to accomplish in such a short time. With simple dietary changes, the Lifestyle Program has successfully cured our patients of hypertension, prediabetes, diabetes, obesity, acid reflux and sleep apnea. Compliance with the Lifestyle Program demonstrates results far superior to any we have seen in terms of the reduction in lipids and sugars and HgbA1c's (the lab test that shows the previous 3-month average glucose or blood sugar levels). More importantly, along with annual savings of $200 to $400 in eliminated prescriptions cost, the only side effects have been: weight loss, clearer thinking, more energy, better sleep, and fewer muscle aches. Oh, yes! Many of our patients have to buy a new wardrobe!

The most common response I get from other doctors when I share my success with *Food as Medicine* is that diets don't work for *their* patients. Hmmm . . . So either their patients have a special, unknown, unique metabolism, or the doctors themselves really don't believe the message—or they don't have a Mike to show their patients how to implement a lifestyle change program.

To be successful, the program must support the patients through the stages of change. Just giving them a handbook is not enough. While not all of the program's elements are covered by insurance plans, we have found that many of the costs associated with a Lifestyle Program are reimbursable. Still, once the patients witness their own results, they are often willing to assume the expenses not covered by insurance, to absorb the cost for "real food". (Real food, incidentally, is not necessarily the most expensive or organically grown.)

I trained as a lipidologist many years ago, which is really a specialty degree in understanding and treating complex lipid disorders, which are very rare by the way. The diseases that we are taught in lipidology I have yet to see in my practice. They are so rare they occur in less than 1 in 5000, so it is very rare that we see these diseases. I started in a lipid clinic in my practice where I would aggressively treat patients' lipids to all the numbers that the guidelines told me to and I learned a few things over the years. One, I was having a hard time getting patients to their goals on these drugs. Number two, these drugs cause enormous side effects. Number three, the drugs weren't making a very big difference in outcomes of whether or not patients would have a heart attack or not or die. The fourth thing I learned was that by actually focusing on their diet and restricting carbohydrates and/or trying to get my patients' carbohydrates as low as possible, their lipid panels improved dramatically, better than with any medication I gave them. I was able to actually stop many of their medications and just continue them on a lifestyle of controlling their carbohydrate intake and their LDL numbers came down, their triglycerides came down, their HDLs rose up, and their sugar levels dropped. Everything I was trying to do with these drugs I was much better at doing with food and better at doing this other thing that Hippocrates said, which was, "First do no harm." I kind of fell into all that and have been doing it ever since.

I have learned that while we human beings can stubbornly adhere to fictions, we are also malleable. With the proper motivation, education and — most important — a therapeutic relationship between patient and practitioner, people want to and will change their dietary habits in order to improve their health. Chronic conditions such as obesity, prediabetes and diabetes cost this country billions of dollars a year, and it gets worse all the time. The answer to our healthcare crisis, in my opinion, is to put 10 lifestyle educators in every primary care medical practice. While I am not sharing *my* Mike, I challenge all physicians, especially primary care physicians, to explore food as medicine.

The underpinnings of our Lifestyle Program are rooted in evidence-based medicine and have been validated repeatedly by lengthy dietary studies done throughout the world. Our program requires patients to minimize the amount of grains (even whole grains), sugars and processed foods they eat each day. Our goal for diabetic patients is to eat less than 75 grams of carbohydrates daily. We don't restrict them from eating red meat, butter and cheese.

We view processed wheat and sugar, not healthy dietary fats, as the enemy. Countless authors of nutritional guidelines have examined the scientific, anthropological and biochemical basis for supporting the conclusion that dietary fats are bad for people but no study has proven it. There have been, however, extremely influential marketing campaigns by the food and pharmaceutical industries that malign fats. Interestingly, there was a time when the American Heart Association supported a low carbohydrate diet that allowed for red meat, butter and cheese. Yet, despite overwhelming evidence to the contrary, the AMA was convinced to adopt the low fat diet as superior.

Having read the studies, books and papers that have been written in the last few decades, we have distilled them into a simple guide of what to eat and what not to eat. Although the ideas contained here may sound novel, they are not. The numerous books in the addendum unveil the myths surrounding the nutritional advice given to us over the last 30 years.

Back in 2002, an article appeared in the New York Times citing the dichotomy of the AMA in refuting the Atkins-type low fat diet yet touting the cause of obesity in this country as being due to a low fat diet[4]. I cite that article as a spark of sanity albeit ignored by our country's widely publicized nutritional guidelines.

Our Guidelines for Healthy Eating

If you're looking for information about how to eat, how to deal with diabetes, and how to maintain your weight, walk right by the magazines and other super market checkout line sources and follow these guidelines:

1. Have a portion of fish, poultry (chicken, turkey, goose, etc) or meat (beef, veal, lamb or pork) with every meal. Wild or grass-fed, organic and hormone-free are best. Don't aim for leaner here; healthy eating isn't about limiting yourself to the leanest; enjoy the fat.
2. Eat eggs frequently; daily would be very good, either at breakfast, as a snack, or in a salad. Choose organic, cage-free and pasture- or grass-fed.
3. Eat a variety of different vegetables throughout the day and week.
4. Occasionally eat nuts or nut butters (remember: peanuts are legumes not nuts, so avoid them and peanut butter as well. Instead, try natural almond and cashew butters.)

---

[4]   *What if it's all been a big fat lie? By Gary Taubes, NY Times July 07, 2002*

5. Depending on your health and weight goals, avoid or greatly reduce all breads, pasta, boxed cereals, and grains — such as brown rice (some white rice is okay), oats, barley, millet, quinoa, buckwheat, amaranth, triticale, etc. Eating two slices of whole wheat bread is no different than eating a candy bar in terms of the effect on blood sugar.

6. Enjoy fats: cook with butter, coconut oil or animal fats; use olive oil and nut oils as much as you want for dressings and as a flavoring (not cooking); don't use products called hydrogenated fats like margarine or Crisco® (originally used as candle material but later remarketed as food); don't use vegetable oil or products with soy oil or seed oils, for example canola.

7. In moderation, use full-fat dairy cream and cheese.

8. Dramatically reduce sweets: desserts, sweetened processed foods; sugar, honey, agave; and dried fruits (which are really no different than a Snicker's® Bar) and candy. Berries are best in the fruit category.

When it comes right down to it, we should all be eating like the diabetic patients in our Lifestyle Program!

THREE: Carbs vs. Fats

If you don't want to become diabetic and don't want to be pre-diabetic, the most powerful thing you can do is limit your carbohydrates to less than 75 gm per day. You may say, well that doesn't sound so hard. Well, if you look at people's diets and if they actually start looking at what they're eating, they are eating anywhere from 150 gm to 300 gm of carbohydrates a day. The human body requires zero carbohydrates to function. Zero. There is no daily minimum requirement of carbohydrates by the human body. We can take fat and protein and synthesize them into carbohydrates as needed. Our body actually prefers fats and ketones to burn and not sugar, but because we are pouring so much sugar in it daily, that is what our bodies have gotten used to burning, but it's not the body's preferred fuel. To prevent diabetes or to cure it or reverse it or control it limit your carbohydrate intake to less than 75 grams daily.

Once your hemoglobin A1c is no longer in diabetic range, in my mind, you are no longer just controlled, you are cured. The way to do that is by taking the old U.S. government food pyramid and turning it upside down. The food pyramid was bought and purchased by all the companies that benefit from being on the base of that pyramid. At the pyramid base are grains as breads, pastas, and cereals. We are told we need a certain number of grains every day and I will tell you that is absolutely not true. We need zero grains for survival. Although there are some grains that are more tolerable, the worst offender in my opinion is the wheat in this country which is a genetically modified grain. Not the wheat of our ancestors, but the wheat that is in most of our current day diets. If you have been diagnosed as prediabetic or diabetic and you eliminate wheat from your diet you will have a dramatic improvement in your blood sugar numbers. You will be able to get off many of your medications.

In terms of people with heart disease, the message of the last 40 years that directs them to adhere to a low-fat diet is not correct. That is a flawed theory and the proof continues to come out showing that it is not correct; that fat is not the enemy.[5][6][7] There are healthy fats, some fats are better for your cellular function than other fats. In the Mediterranean diet which focuses more on adding more olive oil to our diet, other fats are ignored although different fats from nuts are included. My experience has also shown me fat is not the enemy.

I believe that we need naturally occurring fatty meat from healthy animals raised on proper feed. It's not what you eat; it is what the animals have been fed that you're eating. I believe that a cow that is raised on the diet it is supposed to have, which is grass, will have the proper fats in its tissues and if we eat those fats we're fine. If we eat the cow that is raised on grains making their whole fat ratios skewed, we're eating the wrong fats. Although grass-fed beef is more expensive, it contains the right fats. Non-grass-fed beef has the wrong ratios of omega-3 and omega-6 fats in its tissues.

We know from looking at different populations around the world where most of the diet consists of fats, that they have virtually no heart disease compared to us. Firstly, the cattle in those places graze free range. Secondly, the diet of the general world population is mostly based on animal fats either from milk, as among the African Masai whose entire culture depends on cattle, or other animal products such as whale blubber among the Inuit.[8]

---

[5]   *Fat is not the enemy: discovermag.com/2007/may/how-bad-is-fat?*
[6]   *Los Angeles Food Examiner.com*
[7]   *Ezine articles by Keith Lewis*
[8]   *For a more extensive discussion, I recommend reading "Eat Fat; Lose Fat" by Mary Enig*

FOUR: The Cholesterol Story

Cholesterol, which has been maligned for so long, is required in every cell membrane in our body. It insulates all of the neurons in our bodies and our brain, it maintains cellular function, it helps us metabolize vitamins, it helps us produce bile, and it is the precursor of many of our hormones, including our sex hormones. So, we need cholesterol. Cholesterol is not the enemy. If we don't get it in our diets our liver will make it and if we get too much in our diets our liver will make less. So there is a nice little feedback loop that exists in our body.

In the disease atherosclerosis, where you have plaque in your arteries, indeed there is cholesterol in that plaque. But why is it there? Think about this: You are driving home today, or any day, and you see an accident on the side of the road and there are ambulances there helping take care of the victims. Do you think to yourself, oh those ambulances must have caused the accident? No. They are there to help and it is the same thing with cholesterol. Cholesterol is brought to the scene of the crime to help repair the damage that's been done to the artery wall. It is part of the body's repair process. Cholesterol helps form a scab or puts a Band-aid over the injury. What happens after that is that the white cells that rush to anywhere in the body where there is damage don't like the cholesterol being there and they try to remove it causing inflammation.

The take-home message is that cholesterol does not damage the artery wall. It is there as part of the repair process and sometimes the repair process goes awry because there are conditions in the body that are causing inflammation around the injury to the artery so the plaque continues to grow.

Low-fat diets actually make things worse and have not been of any benefit in the last 40 years. It turns out that the healthier diet is the low-carb diet not the low-fat one.

Bottom line: high cholesterol itself is not always a disease, it is just a number. It is not a disease unless you have a cholesterol of 500 or 600. Then you have one of these complicated, inherited, genetic cholesterol diseases which change the whole story. The majority of people do not have these diseases although they may have an elevated cholesterol number. That is not good or bad, it just is a number.

The general belief is that if you have high cholesterol you are more likely to have heart disease. In actuality, if you look at people who are admitted to the hospital with a heart attack, half of them have normal cholesterol or normal LDL so how can you say a disease is caused by high cholesterol when half of the people that have the disease have normal cholesterol? It's one of the best propagated myths I have ever seen and it continues today. So, don't focus so much on your numbers unless you already actually have atherosclerosis. If you do have atherosclerosis then, yes, your doctor should be looking at your numbers trying to keep the amount of LDL particles lower so that the plaque does not continue to grow. But most people don't have the disease, they just have high cholesterol. Their doctors are prescribing medicine based on a number instead of looking further to see if they have a disease that merits medication. In fact, as recently as November of 2013, the latest and greatest new guidelines were released by the American Heart Association and American College of Cardiology, and they support *broadening* the use of statins

These new fangled guidelines (once again, admitting that 50% plus of what we know is and was wrong) do away almost with the old reliance on LDL cholesterol levels. Instead, the decision to go on a statin is now based upon risk levels. And guess what? The experts lowered the risk level criteria so millions of people that were previously considered healthy are now labeled as diseased, eligible for lifelong statin therapy. The latest guidelines for statin therapy use a new complex risk calculator which overestimates risk thus bringing more healthy people under the umbrella of illness.

Here are the current recommended guidelines for statin therapy (Remember these guidelines change as the wind does.):

1) People with no cardiovascular disease between the ages of 40-75 with a 7.5% or higher risk for having a heart attack or stroke within 10 years
2) People 21 or older with an LDL equal to or greater than 190 mg/dL
3) All people with Type I and Type 2 diabetes ages 40-75
4) People with a history of a cardiovascular event

Now I have no problem or argument with number 4. These people have a disease and should be treated. The other 3 groups are in enormous grey zones with room for debate which I leave to others more educated than I to address. The crux of the matter, in my opinion, is that much if not all cardiovascular risk calculators are just surrogate measurements of a person's age. If you take any combination of risk factors and plug them into the calculator, you will see that simply changing the age has an enormous impact on the resultant risk number.

For example: an otherwise healthy 40 year old white man, who doesn't smoke, doesn't have diabetes or high blood pressure, and has a cholesterol of 200, and an HDL of 40 has a calculated 1% risk of having a heart attack in the next 10 years. So this guy is left alone. However if you make him 65 years old and change nothing else he now has an 11.4% risk and needs to be on a statin for the remainder of his life. Regardless of any other risk factor, according to the current guidelines, you can count on a life sentence of taking statins.

I look forward to seeing all sorts of crazy, unintended consequences of these new guidelines. Remember in 5 years when we get another new set of guidelines, it will be accompanied by the words "we were wrong again". Stay tuned

---

Posted September 24, 2012: **Living in Wellness**

When I think of *Living in Wellness* I think about living a balanced life: emotionally, socially, nutritionally, intellectually, occupationally, physically, environmentally and spiritually. I think of *Living in Wellness* as life that is fundamentally lived in a way that is of benefit to others.

However, I have noticed that for many patients the goal isn't wellness, but to live longer. And, not just longer, but almost without aging. For most people the goal in going to the gym and working out is to extend life not to be well for the time they live. Their goal in taking care of their hearts and lungs isn't to live fully engaged, peaceful and loving lives, but to ensure longevity!

Living in wellness is about understanding how to live with who we are in body and mind in a way that is present and fully engaged. Being here, being aware, being present to what is, and acting appropriately, is wellness. When we are here, when we are aware and engaged, we always act in ways that benefit us, our families and our friends, colleagues and community. We are peaceful and loving rather than stressed and anxious. We respond appropriately, for example, to medical conditions and test results by looking clearly at our options and choosing the one that is best for us and those around us.

Living in wellness, when we have a cold, we realize we don't need to be upset about having to blow our nose; wellness is simply doing it; responding to what is happening without writing a story that says "I'm sick," "I hate having a cold," or "I always get colds when work is the busiest."

Many patients with Type One diabetes give themselves insulin shots daily all their lives and never think of themselves as "sick." Just as in the morning when they get up and their body tells them to shower and brush their teeth, in the evening their body tells them to inject themselves without making it into a story. I believe this is the model for living in the best, most effective way; what I call living in the state of wellness is living the good life.

Wellness is the state of mind that arises spontaneously, almost always without our noticing, so long as we are not telling ourselves we are sick. This isn't about denying a medical condition; it isn't about ignoring symptoms. It is simply responding appropriately without thinking it should be otherwise. That is, without saying, "I was never like this before. This shouldn't be happening to me." Wellness isn't about comparing ourselves to how we were 20 or 30 or 40 years ago; it is about simply allowing ourselves to be here now, present to who we are this moment and responding with patience and caring.

Ironically, when things are "going right," we never think to ourselves, "Wow, I've been well all day today. What a blessing." Yet the moment we sneeze twice in a row, or learn about a "high" number on a blood test, all we can think is "I'm sick", "This isn't me," or "If I can just get the numbers down, then everything will be all right again" (meaning, "So I can go on to live forever.")

In my experience, patients want and need to collaborate in all aspects of their health not just find and get proper medical care. They want and need information and suggestions, explanation, and practical guidelines, and they want and need the clarity of reflective and contemplative practices that will bring balance into their lives. This is the way people can then live comfortably and well.

I believe *Living in Wellness* is what happens when we stop attributing false meanings and values to normal bodily processes, like aging. *Living in Wellness* is coming to the realization of how to live life. I offer you the information you need in order to be *Living in Wellness*.

FIVE: HDL and LDL What's Fat Got To Do With It?

HDL and LDL are not fats they are lipoproteins, which are the form in which our body can move cholesterol and fats through our bloodstream. When you eat a fatty meal the fat is routed to the liver. From the fats our liver then creates these lipoproteins (lipo means fat) that are released into the bloodstream. As fats they are not soluble in blood; as fatty proteins they are.

LDL has been demonized and HDL glorified. This is the result of simple minds telling a story and if you tell a story long enough people grow to believe it. During World War 2 the minister of propaganda for the Nazi party, Joseph Goebbels, was fond of saying that if you tell a lie big enough and keep repeating it, people will eventually come to believe it. Big pharma and big food and big government all know that the bigger the lie the more people are willing to unquestioningly accept it. That is what's happened with LDL and HDL. We have been told that LDL is the enemy and HDL is the good guy and it's a nice story, it sounds good. People love a story of good vs. evil. But that's just not the case. Our body doesn't work like that; it's not how we were designed.

LDL is the deliverer of cholesterol and fat to our bodies. Every cell in our body needs cholesterol and fat in order to survive.

Once we start realizing that LDL is not the enemy, we start looking at types of LDL. There is big LDL, there's little LDL. It turns out the little LDL is a little worse than the big LDL. What causes the little LDL, the small dense LDL? Once again, it is driven by diet and what we eat. The more carbohydrates we eat, the more small dense LDL we make. If you believe in the LDL theory that big is better, then you want to avoid carbohydrates and you will have nice big, fluffy, bouncy LDL that can't penetrate into that clean-up repair zone. It doesn't matter what your LDL number is as much as its particle size. Is there a measure for that?

You can pretty much tell what kind of particle size and number the patient has by simple observation. Just looking at the patient's belly size I can predict pretty closely what their LDL particle size and number are. If someone's belly enters the exam room before the patient does, I can tell that they are going to have a very big particle

17

number and they are going to have small, dense particle size. Which one is more important? The answer is: it depends.

It depends on what company is doing the study. Just like sub-sects of a religion, either particle number is more important or the particle size is more important. If particle size is the important criteria (as it was in 2010), there are ways to test for it. One test is called NMR testing, another is called VAP testing, there is also another test called Berkley testing. But again, a look at the patient will give me a good estimate of their carbohydrate intake and the corresponding LDL particle number. The size of their belly will alert me to the size of the LDL particle. Big belly? The particles are going to be small and dense with a low HDL and high triglyceride number. Based on my 25 years of treating patients with high cholesterol and high blood pressure, in my opinion the only patients that should be checked for particle size are those who actually have plaque in their arteries—atherosclerosis—and who are being monitored for treatment.

The triglyceride number is mostly a surrogate marker of a person's carbohydrate intake. If you eat a lot of sugar you are going to have a high triglyceride level. If you restrict sugar you will have a low triglyceride number and a high HDL. This is true in the great majority of humans. HDL is also usually a very good marker of saturated fat intake. We've been afraid of eating saturated fats because we've been told that fat is the enemy and, again, we have recently learned that, oh, we're wrong on that one.

The accepted story goes on to say that HDL works like a garbage truck. That it insinuates itself into the artery wall, sucks up cholesterol, and brings it back to the liver to dump it out like a dump truck. Lipidologists love telling that story when they give talks about how HDL works. Unfortunately, it's a little more complicated.

When you're told that your HDL is low, ask, "Will it matter if I raise it? Will that change my life expectancy? Will that make me have fewer heart attacks?" Here is what we learned: when we got peoples' LDL number down using statins, we were able to decrease their risk of having a heart attack by a whopping 1%-2%! The statistical risk was lowered but the absolute risk not. A lot of people continue to have heart attacks. Well, what else can we go after? How about HDL?

There is a correlation between low HDL and heart attacks. So the thought ran: maybe if we raise the HDL number people won't have heart attacks or die anymore. HDL became the new drug target. Drugs to elevate HDL were developed. Again, it was all theory that if we were to raise HDL we would decrease heart attacks and we would improve peoples' life spans. This is why billions of dollars have been spent to develop these HDL elevating drugs.

Let me digress. There are always exceptions to a rule and especially when the rule is wrong. Here's an example: In the Italian village Limone sul Garda, 3.5% of the population have a mutation of one of the proteins found on human HDL. This mutant protein is named ApoA-1 Milano and its presence was associated with reduced cardiovascular disease even though the protein causes low HDL and elevated triglycerides. So, going along with the popular theory, in the early 2000s a pharmaceutical company called Esperion began synthesizing an ApoA-1 Milano product to infuse into our arteries. Pfizer bought the company for nearly a billion dollars. Some time later in the early 2000s, Pfizer went on to sell the rights for ApoA-1 Milano to the Medicines Company for a fraction of what they had paid Esperion. Currently no drugs based on ApoA-1 Milano are commercially available. I leave it to you to decide why Pfizer would have sold such a potentially valuable drug.

We also have other HDL elevating drugs that we have had for a long time. Niacin as Niaspan® is one which we know raises HDL very well. I used to actually speak for a drug company that produced Niaspan. I confess to being brainwashed into believing that niacin did all these amazing things, not only to the numbers but to the plaque itself and that people would then live longer. But, lo and behold, that theory was blown out of the water in the last year or so.

The National Heart Lung Blood Institute, or NHLBI, did a study which was called the Aim High Study.[9] They stopped the study in May of 2011. The study was to answer the question of whether or not raising HDL in people who had some disease would lower the rate of their dying of a heart attack or of a stroke or of something related to cardiovascular disease. These people were already on a statin and half of them were given Niaspan and the other half given a placebo and they were followed for a few years. They stopped the trial early because they saw that there was absolutely no statistical or clinical

---

[9]   www.NIH.gov/news/health/may2011/nilbi-26.htm

significance, no difference between the two arms of the study. The people were dying of heart attacks or strokes and actually, when they broke it down and looked at the details, there actually were more people that were having a certain type of stroke that were taking niacin. That was a huge trial that was sponsored by our government to look at and answer this question and it answered it. It said, no – there is no difference whatsoever. There is no good reason patients should take niacin or any other HDL elevating drug.

I can raise your HDL, I can lower your triglycerides, I can lower your LDL I can do all these with a drug, but it's not going to a make a difference in your life whatsoever. You are not going to live longer, you're still going to have a heart attack or a stroke, but you are going to have great numbers. It's as if I could take your diseased lawn and paint it green; you would have a beautiful-looking lawn, but it's not going to change the underlying condition of your lawn. Your lawn would still be sick and diseased, but it would look good. The Aim High Study confirmed that.

To put an end to the niacin and HDL story, Merck then came out with an announcement regarding another niacin-type drug.[10] They studied 26,000 people who took the drug and after 3.9 years the outcome was that it made no difference whatsoever. The current evidence in 2013 is that putting patients on niacin will not reduce their cardiovascular disease risk. So that's it with niacin.

Then we had these other drugs, which were very fancy drugs which also raised HDL. They did it by inhibiting an enzyme called cholesterol ester transfer protein (CETP). These CETP inhibitors dramatically increased HDL. These drugs can get HDL up by 70% and lower LDL by 30%. So, this was an amazing drug that Pfizer spent another billion on for developing and testing. It turned out, lo and behold, more people were dying by taking this drug than not taking it. So once again, that drug never made it to market.

So, the take-home message is if you do not have heart disease, if you've never had a heart attack and you've never had a stroke, you really should not be so worried about your LDL and HDL. You shouldn't be worried about anything because worry doesn't change the outcome. But if you want to stay healthy and enjoy the life you

---

[10]   www.reuters.com/article/2013/03/09/us-heart-niacin-merck...

have while you're alive, then you should really be focusing on eating real foods, which probably brings us to the next question that I would ask if I were you, "Well what about the Mediterranean diet?"

Posted blog: **Eating for Wellness**

Nutrition is one of the key components of *Living in Wellness*, yet it isn't often explained clearly. In fact, recently as I was thumbing through a cooking magazine for diabetics, I realized that more often than not people are likely to get bad or wrong information, even from the most apparently trustworthy sources.

So let me state this clearly: For good health and weight maintenance limit your dietary carbohydrates to 50 to 75 grams/day. In plain English, that's a low carb diet. Indeed, the Type 2 diabetic and pre-diabetic patients I treat have effectively prevented or reversed/cured their condition by limiting their dietary intake of carbohydrates to less than 50 grams/day. And many of my patients have seen results within as little as 4 weeks! No medication prescribed to-date can claim the same.

My rule for a healthy lifestyle diet is this: if the serving size has more than 12g of carbohydrates, it's a dessert. Minimize, share or eliminate desserts. If you are monitoring nutrition labels and see that there are more than 12 g of carbohydrates in a food product, it is most likely processed and should be avoided. In fact, if you stick to protein, healthy fats and veggies you won't need to count or worry about carbs.

SIX: The Mediterranean Diet

The Mediterranean diet[11] is as good, if not better, than being on a statin. It is rich in real food, non-processed foods, vegetables, fish, nuts, the normal oils that we should be eating that are real oils – not processed or created in a laboratory. Aside from olive oil and nuts, it consists mostly of animal-based foods. People on this diet are not just eating lean cuts of meat; they eat pretty much the organ meats, the liver, and the heart, all of the parts of that animal. Most of the animal does not go to waste in Mediterranean countries. Please note that they eat animal fats yet have less heart disease and thereby are living longer than we are. It is our food supply that is ridiculously sick so if you can somehow get back to eating as close to real food as possible, that is, know where your food is raised and who is raising it and/or do it yourself, you're going to be way better off.

When modified by removing the whole grains, the Mediterranean Diet is, in my opinion, the ultimate anti-inflammatory eating plan. It is rich in anti-inflammatory omega fats, heart-healthy mono-unsaturated fats and low in sugar. A study called the Lyon Diet Heart Study focused on men with risk factors for heart disease. They put the men on either a diet low in saturated fat and cholesterol or on a Mediterranean Diet which is rich in omega-3s from fish and mono-unsaturated fats from nuts and olive oil. The study was terminated early. There was a 70% reduction in heart attacks in the group that ate the Mediterranean Diet. Of note is that there was no change in these men's LDL cholesterol levels at all. So, it's the inflammation, my friends, not the LDL cholesterol level that matters. Diets high in sugars (carbohydrates) and processed foods contribute to inflammation. Eating a Mediterranean diet without the whole grains seems to be of great benefit.

If I'm asked what I think about the wine in that diet, here's my answer: If you already drink wine, follow the diet's recommendations. If you don't drink wine, don't begin drinking wine just to stick to the diet.

I'd also want people to keep in mind that the Mediterranean lifestyle is different from ours. People there actually walk. We drive.

---

[11]   www.nejm.org/doi/full...

We drive to dinner and we drive home. They walk and stroll pretty much most of their evening both before and after dinner.

But, promising though it is, it's my feeling that the Mediterranean diet is destined to disappear from the Earth. America has introduced and marketed our processed fast foods to the rest of the world and because of the convenience they promise, the seduction of the carbohydrates offered, and their low price, a Mediterranean diet is very soon going to be hard to stick to anywhere on our globe.

SEVEN: Risk Factors and What They Mean to You

When deciding to take a medicine for the rest of your life, there needs to be a conversation between you and your doctor. If the doctor gets huffy and gets defensive ("How dare you ask me that?") then that patient-doctor relationship is flawed and it's time to look for a different doctor. If the doctor is not willing to have a heart-to-heart (no pun intended) conversation with the patient about their heart and arterial health, then what's the point of that relationship? It is more of a power relationship where the doctor is saying, "Here take this, I know best," and apparently the doctor doesn't always know best because, as we have discovered from hospital statistics[12], the doctor is wrong 50% of the time or science changes. If the doctor doesn't read new and old studies critically or does not know how to interpret the studies and just goes to meetings and listens to the so-called experts, it's time to change doctors.

The so-called experts are for the most part on salary from drug companies. In fact, most of the doctors involved in these expert panels that create guidelines are on the payroll of the drug companies. They are biased towards the drugs and if they say otherwise they are lying to themselves. These guideline writers or creators are, in my opinion, inherently biased. (Eight out of ten of the expert panelists that handed down the last set of guidelines to us simpletons had financial ties to the pharmaceutical industry). Can these experts ever be conflict-free? I think not! Even severing ties with industry while working on or creating new guidelines and promising not to have any industry ties for 2 years after the guidelines are published does not abolish the conflict. That's mere window dressing. So, if you cannot have the heart-to-heart about your heart with your doctor, I am not saying come see me. I'm not looking for more patients. I am saying find the doctor with whom you can have the conversation about risk and real numbers.

Risk is an interesting word. It is a statistical word. There are numerous risk factors. There are probably 100 different risk factors for developing heart disease. A risk factor for heart disease means that someone did a mathematical study of the association between one thing and another and they determined that, for example, more people with gray hair have heart disease than people with no gray

---

[12]   www.sciencedaily.com/releases/2009/01...

hair. So, gray hair becomes a risk factor. It does not mean it's the cause. Risk factors and cause are completely different. We have confused matters to the point that when people have been told they have a risk factor or even two or three risk factors, they believe they actually have the disease. That's not the case. What they have is this correlation. Again, they have gray hair, they're old, and so they have two risk factors for having heart disease. If I modify that risk factor, if I dye that patient's hair black, that would not decrease their risk of having a heart attack. The risk factor is there but it is not the same as having the condition; the correlations are indeed there but that is not a diagnosis. Often times the correlations we look at are not the right ones. What risk factors do I look at as the most diagnostically important?

The big belly. I can't miss that risk factor. That is a risk factor for many reasons. The biggest one being that that belly, when too big, almost turns into its own organ, its own endocrine organ that starts secreting all sorts of chemicals, toxins, and cytokines which are triggering proteins that send inflammatory messages to the immune system creating even more inflammation. The cause of atherosclerosis or heart disease is the result of damage made to the inner artery wall. Inflammation damages a lot of inner walls. People with big bellies have these pro-inflammatory factories going that need to be shut down. So that's a big risk factor; you can't miss that one.

The second risk factor is high blood pressure and we can easily lower high blood pressure. Since most of the time that big belly is from carbohydrate intake, when you restrict people's carbohydrates their bellies go away and their blood pressure goes down.

The third risk factor I look at is obvious. Does the patient smoke? We know that smokers have more heart disease than nonsmokers. Why is that? It's because of the smoke that damages the artery wall. It's not the nicotine, it's the smoke. It's the 500 plus different toxins and ingredients in the smoke. You should not be breathing in smoke of any sort. So smoking is a big one.

Then I look at some tests. What are the patient's sugar levels? What is their hemoglobin A1c number? This test shows what the sugar levels have been averaging for 90 days, not just one day. If someone comes to the doctor, they are fasting and they have a sugar of 95 they think great, it's below 100, I'm fine. But people don't live in a fasting state. The hemoglobin A1c tells me what their sugars have averaged for 90 days and I can tell you from 25 years of experience that people with diabetes and/or pre-diabetes get more heart disease than other people no matter what their cholesterol is. That is a correlation—a big risk factor—and so I always look at their hemoglobin A1c.

Lastly, I look at their family history. If they had parents or siblings who died young, in their 30s and 40s, they may have a rare inherited lipid abnormality that should be investigated further. It is also possible the whole family was exposed to an infection that caused damage to their inner arterial walls.

Those are the big risk factors I look at. Not so much the lipid panel. For determining risk, the lipid panel to me is as good as flipping a coin. As risk factors go, the results of the lipid panel tests are 50-50. As I've said above, 50% of the people that have heart attacks have normal cholesterol. So looking at their lipid panel is not a critical risk factor; the ones I've listed are: Size of belly, blood pressure, smoking, blood sugar levels and family history.

A lot of people labor under the idea that they can wait until they are actually diabetic and only then deal with it. But, if you've ever seen an iceberg (I don't know how many people have seen icebergs), but what they see of the iceberg is the tip of the iceberg that is sticking up above the surface of the water. They are seeing about maybe 3% to 5% of that iceberg, but below the water that iceberg is enormous. It's like a giant pyramid and all they are seeing is the top of the pyramid sticking out of the water. So underneath the surface of the water the iceberg is enormous. It's the same thing in pre-diabetes. This person can look fine on the surface, but underneath the surface their metabolic health is being attacked daily. They have sugar sticking to all the proteins in their body and they are causing damage to their kidneys, to their nerves, to all of their arteries, to their eyes, to their – to everything – while we're waiting for this number to become diabetic. I get concerned when I see a HgbA1c level of 5.7 and I intervene and say we have to do something right now. If the doctor and patient do nothing, it is more than likely the patient will continue to drift along towards full blown diabetes. All the time experiencing cellular damage as (s)he waits.

Posted blog: *Living in Wellness with a Serious Illness*

Regardless of how right or wrong we believe we are about health and treatment, about cholesterol and statins, about diabetes and diet, about smoking and cancer, at some point most of us will have to deal with a serious, life-threatening illness. It is then, more than ever before, that we will need to understand how to live in wellness.

Living in Wellness is about your frame of mind. It is living in a way that is aware of what's happening in your body and allowing yourself to be fully engaged with it. Being fully present and engaged with the body means you are responding appropriately to the conditions of your body, to a serious illness if that's what is present, but without asking it to be other than what it is, without judging it or evaluating it or wanting it not to be. In other words, responding to it without denying that it needs attention and without making it worse for ourselves with fear and worry and stress.

When we learn to see the preciousness of each moment, when we learn to cherish each and every moment and each and every living being, then whether we have a cold or cancer does not become a source of stress and anxiety. Of course we respond to the cold or the cancer, or any other condition, but we respond from the awareness of a need to be a caretaker: one who cares for our own well-being, which boils down to also caring for our families and friends, and so on.

To become fully engaged, we start by being mindful. Being mindful simply means being present with what we are and with what is happening, without judgment. If it is ADD or ADHD or PTSD, or HIV/AIDS or diabetes or cancer, *Living in Wellness* tells us to be aware of the condition, to respond to it appropriately with whatever treatment or procedure is best. *Living in Wellness* is about process and peacefulness, not stress and outcome. If we undertake the best treatment we can, for any medical condition, it will result in the best outcome. However, if we focus on the outcome, we will increase our stress and lack the clarity needed to make informed best choices. What we do not do, however, when we are *Living in Wellness*, is to create more tension and stress around the condition by writing stories like "This shouldn't be" and "Why me? It's unfair" and "I hate myself like this." Those complicate the situation, make us more upset, and prevent us from seeing clearly the appropriate response for the condition.

Living in Wellness reminds us not to get hung up on the labels and the letters or even the numbers. *Living in Wellness* reminds us that the meaning in life comes from awareness of our inner peaceful nature and from responding to ourselves and others, responding to the world from that place. Learning to live in wellness takes time and patience and motivation, especially in the face of a serious medical condition. But it pays off. So where does one start?

Listening to a guided body scan meditation each night before bed (a side effect of which will be to relax you and help you sleep better) is an easy and excellent place in which to begin a *Living in Wellness* practice. During a body scan meditation, you are guided to visualize each part of the body, notice the sensations there, and to breathe into them, allowing them to soften and relax. Doing a body scan meditation each night gradually heightens your awareness and makes you more and more mindful.

Over a period of days and weeks, this new way of seeing yourself extends out into the world; you spontaneously trade judgment for awareness, stress for peacefulness. You see the world with an open heart, rather than an anxious mind, and you respond in a way that is appropriate, caring and comfortable for all involved.

There is no doubt that this is a big shift in the way we normally process information. But at some point, we realize that the other option, to continue to process information in ways that make us uneasy and uncomfortable and stressed, just doesn't make sense any longer.

Living in wellness also means being mindful of what you eat. If you need it simple here's the cheat sheet:

Don't Eat This

Remember It's all about the sugar (sugar = fat, diabetes, inflammation, heart disease, arthritis, and a host of diseases)

1. *No Grains* – grains are the largest contributing factor to pre-diabetes, diabetes and abnormal weight gain and obesity, in the form of rice, *all* breads (yes, that means no whole wheat or multi-grain or sprouted or otherwise healthfully touted); oatmeal (definitely not oatmeal...not even steel-cut oats); not any type of boxed cereal; pizza, bakery goods or pasta; no granola bars or protein bars (all contain wheat or corn syrup; corn's a grain and grains makes you gain fat and cause inflammation). Living without grain is not as difficult as you think.
2. *No beans*
3. *Limit fruit* to 1 serving of fruit daily. No fruit daily is OK.
4. *No fruit juices*, Gatorade®, Red Bull®, energy drinks, no diet or regular soft drinks
5. *No milk* – no low-fat or reduced fat dairy products (a little whole fat cheese, unflavored yogurt or cream in moderation)
6. *No potato chips or fries* — no way
7. *No artificial sweeteners*, that includes Truvia®, NuStevia®, or In the Raw®. If you must, pure stevia extract is acceptable in small amounts.
8. *Don't buy anything that's low fat (low fat = high sugar, and your body needs the fat)*
9. *Don't buy anything diet or "lite" (that usually means it is sweetened with artificial sweeteners)*

EIGHT: More Questions to Ask Your Doctor

If you are on a statin drug, have a conversation with your doctor. The conversation should go something like this:

"Doctor, I understand I have high cholesterol and that's why you prescribed the statin for me, but please tell me the absolute benefit to me from being on this drug. How much is the statin going to decrease my personal risk of a) having a heart attack and b) dying?"

He should be able to answer you straight out.

"Ms. Jones, your absolute risk reduction of being on the statin is anywhere from 1% to 3% so what that means is by being on the statin I can decrease your risk of having a heart attack over the next five years by 1%. That's why you are on the statin."

Now, it's important you know that prescribing a drug in order to prevent some event or condition is called primary prevention. We are trying to prevent the first event of a heart attack or a stroke or something like that. There is also what we call secondary prevention, which is prescribing a drug to someone who already has had a heart attack or stroke to reduce the risk of their having another such event. These people do better on statins. The data is better for secondary prevention. If you've already had a heart attack or a stroke and you are on a statin you do get a better benefit from that statin than someone who is on it to prevent the first event. So don't just stop your statins without talking to your physician first.

Now ask: "Am I on this drug as a primary prevention strategy or as secondary prevention? If I'm taking it as a primary prevention strategy, is there another way I can lower my risk by that little 1%? Is there something else I could do instead of taking this drug?"

Ask: "What are the side effects of statins?"

As I've noted above, the side effects are well documented. Those are well-known beyond what the package insert warnings state and are only what were observed during the drug trial, not what's been gathered since the drugs have been on the market and millions more patients exposed to them. Your doctor would say the biggest side effects of statins are muscle aches that can be quite incapacitating and once you stop the statin those muscle aches stop. Number two, you can have joint aches. Number three, you can have memory disturbances. There are reports of people who have had complete amnesia. There are people who are diagnosed with dementia actually caused by the use of statins. Statins can raise your blood sugars and actually cause diabetes. Those are the big side effects. We can mitigate those side effects; we can decrease the risk of the muscle aches and the joint aches. We can put people on CoQ10 and we can maximize their vitamin D levels, but again this is what is done for people who really need to be on statins. Out of 100 people taking statins probably 1 or 2 of them really need to be on the drug. The other 98 or 99 have been prescribed it as a knee-jerk reaction by physicians treating a number, not willing to really look and see if the patient has a condition meriting the treatment and/or is going to get benefit from the drug. And not examining the patient and assessing whether he would gain the same benefit from eating real foods and eating differently than taking a drug for the rest of their lives.

I tell physicians they need to give their patients the choice. I do. I sit across the desk from my patients, I show them their numbers, and then I pull out the piece of paper that says this is what the statin will do. I can lower your risk of having a heart attack by this percent, I can lower your risk of having a stroke by this percent, I can affect your total mortality by this percent – you can either go on the medications OR we can work on your lifestyle and I can teach you how to eat properly and get the same benefit you would have gotten from that drug by eating real foods and proper foods.

Most people, given the chance and after being educated as to the real numbers, say, "Are you crazy doctor? For a 1% chance I'm not going to take this drug for the rest of my life!" And they choose to let food be their medicine.

Posted blog: **Eating for Health and Weight Loss**

With a myriad of health and wellness diet choices available, in my Lifestyle Program we have blended the best of an Atkins, low-carb and "Paleo" way of eating. For more than 4 years, many thousands of our patients have achieved exceptional health and healthy weight-loss by following our recommended food plan.

This lifestyle way of eating is based on both science and evidence. The habits our healthy ancestors gave us are a good framework for discovering what our food really does to our bodies. Adopting those habits can also demonstrate how to live the most vital lives. Our ancestors ate the whole spectrum of animal-source food (beef, fish, shellfish, poultry, pork, lamb, bison, etc.) including animal fat and organs, eggs, and vegetables but only limited amounts of fruits and nuts.

On the other hand, some foods that we started eating about 10,000 years ago in the beginning of the agricultural revolution are completely alien to our metabolisms. These foods wreak havoc in our bodies, often causing obesity, Type 2 diabetes, hypertension, heart disease, autoimmune diseases, osteoporosis, Alzheimer's and a host of other conditions that were unknown to our ancestors until then and that plague us today.

Some of the worst offenders in today's American diet are actually government-recommended, because bad science and economic agendas have demonized foods such as saturated fat, cholesterol and red meat. We should be eliminating from our diet grain products, excess sugar, vegetable seed oils, legumes and dairy, most of which are cited in the United States government-sponsored food pyramid (or "plate" recently) as healthy.

NINE: The Breakfast Story

Among the things we've learned is that our patients have difficulty figuring out what to have for breakfast after we advise them to eliminate most traditional breakfast foods.

Living in Wellness requires us to power up with protein, and breakfast is where this starts each day. Eggs, meat, poultry and fish need to become the mainstay of our morning meal, not oatmeal, boxed cereal and bread. There is absolutely no need for any carbohydrates in the morning (unless you happen to be running a marathon before going to the office).

Although the practice is ingrained (no pun intended) to have cereal and bread for breakfast, the fact is that grains are just plain bad for us. Amazing as it may seem, as an overarching rule: there are no healthy cereals. Alan Watson's *Cereal Killer* is a great book about this. Just remember, the human body requires ZERO grams of ingested carbohydrates to function. That's right, ZERO.

There is compelling evidence that virtually everything the experts have told us for the past four decades about obesity, diabetes, and weight loss is wrong. We need to be cutting down the carbs while powering up the protein. Not the other way around, which is what our government and dieticians have mistakenly been telling us for the past 40 years.

Structurally, eating well at breakfast is very difficult, not only for my patients but for me and my family as well. While I know absolutely and unequivocally that breakfast should be no different from any other meal, telling my 10-year-old son that we're having leftover roast beef and broccoli for breakfast just doesn't cut it. I might get away with corned-beef hash made with sweet potatoes, but he hates corned beef; God knows I've tried. He wants oatmeal and boxed cereal, and so does my daughter.

I do not believe that oatmeal has any health benefits. In fact, it raises blood sugars in a dramatic and unhealthy way. Please stop watching TV ads (I wish I could get my kids to do that too!) for these products. The few, big companies that make oatmeal and breakfast cereals do not have your best interests in mind. I do.

It seems our entire breakfast world is made up of cereals, breads, bagels and muffins. Once you eliminate these foods from your life, what is left? Yogurt, right? Wrong. Most yogurts are actually dessert treats because they have more than 20g of sugar in them. If you want yogurt it needs to be a full-fat, low-carb yogurt (less than 12g of carbohydrates), which fortunately can still be found in most supermarkets.

In reality, there is a plethora of food options for breakfast. It just requires some thinking, preparation and, oh yeah, mindfulness.

Let's start with eggs. Eggs are the perfect nutritious food. They will not kill you; they don't raise your cholesterol and cause heart attacks. Most of us (95%) can eat 8 eggs a day and not even see a rise in our blood cholesterol levels! That may not be what the government is saying, but it is the truth.

So I urge you to increase your egg intake, with one caveat. Eat real eggs from chickens that are grass fed. Why? Because they are healthier eggs with a better balance of fats and nutrients.

Egg packaging is very deceptive; if the carton doesn't say "free-range" don't buy it. *Whole Foods* sells free-range eggs. Forget about all the other phrases, like cage-free and organic and vegetarian-fed and omega-3 added. The only thing that counts is "free-range." Eat these eggs any way you want: scrambled, poached, fried, soft-boiled. Eat them often; they are good for you. Try hard-boiling a dozen on Sunday night and grabbing a couple on your way out the door every morning if you have to eat on the run. If you have no other option but McDonalds, order a bacon or sausage and egg biscuit and throw out the biscuit.

Leftover cooked chicken, fish, and beef are ideal for powering up with protein in the morning. For a quick breakfast, toss half a cup of leftover chicken, fish or beef into two beaten free-range eggs. Melt a tablespoon or so of butter in a non-stick skillet, add the eggs and meat and stir continuously until the eggs scramble to the texture you want: soft and creamy or firm. Season them with salt and pepper.

You might want to top the eggs with some fresh herbs (like tarragon or parsley), or with some *salsa* or *salsa verde*, with some sliced avocados or guacamole, or with some leftover tomato sauce. You can add a tablespoon or so of curry or chili powder to the eggs to heighten the flavors. It's a great quick breakfast.

One of my patients, Carrie, has discovered delicious non-carb fake oatmeal I love. If you just can't give up the idea of cereals, eat this every day. To make 2 servings of Carrie's "oatmeal:" in a large bowl, whisk together 3 egg whites, 1 cup almond or coconut milk, 1½ tablespoons flaxseed meal (available in most supermarkets) 1 mashed ripe banana, ½ cup coarsely chopped nuts (almonds, cashews, walnuts, pecans, whichever is your favorite), 1 teaspoon ground cinnamon, ½ teaspoon vanilla extract. Transfer to a medium-size saucepan and cook over medium heat, stirring continuously, until hot and thick, just a couple of minutes. Serve immediately.

Sarah Fragaso's *Everyday Paleo Recipes for Life* (available online) is a good source for recipes and wonderful breakfast ideas. Surf around the site when you have a few free minutes.

Making the switch to a healthy diet can seem hard at first, but with time, it will become easier and easier. Just remember, historically, grains were introduced into our diets recently in our evolution toward civilization and they've caused us, and continue to cause us, trouble in the form of autoimmune diseases, digestive disorders, and a host of other ailments.

TEN: Final Words

I like to advise my patients to stay skeptical. There is a commercial that my son loves; it's a beer commercial about the most interesting man in the world. At the end of it the man says, "Stay thirsty my friends." So I would say to everyone—patients and physicians alike—stay skeptical my friends of what we're taught.

My overriding belief is that of the ancient Greek physician, Hippocrates. He said, "Let food be thy medicine." This is as true today as it was back in the 4th century BC. Like him, I believe that the way to regain balance in health is by going back to basics and eating properly. So when I say more education, less medication I mean it really is important to talk to patients and spend time educating them as to how their current diet is causing most of their medical problems. If they are educated and shown the light, if you will, and are allowed to make changes that their physician helps them make, they can dramatically improve their health and forego medications. Most prescribed medications, if you look at the package insert, advise that diet and exercise should be tried first, but patients do neither because no physician has the time to sit and teach their patients what to eat. Then there is the issue that most doctors don't even know what to advise their patients to eat since nutritional guidelines change all the time.

In medical school they say to all the new medical students on their first day, "50% of what we teach you now is wrong and we don't know which half it is." That's a pretty powerful statement. Doctors have known this for years. The iconic physician, Sir William Osler,[13] said, "The philosophies of one age have become the absurdities of the next, and the foolishness of yesterday has become the wisdom of tomorrow." Medical facts are continually being disproven yet it

---

[13] **Sir William Osler, 1st Baronet** (July 12, 1849 – December 29, 1919) was a Canadian physician and one of the four founding professors of Johns Hopkins Hospital. Osler created the first residency program for specialty training of physicians, and he was the first to bring medical students out of the lecture hall for bedside clinical training. He is known as the "Father of Modern Medicine".

fascinates me that so often we believe so dogmatically in what we are told, we are afraid to let it go.

I'm ending with what I opened and that is to stay skeptical, be your own advocate, do your own research, don't believe me, don't believe the experts, do your homework, and then have a conversation with your physician. Let's not focus so much on this scary thing that is going to happen 40-50 years from now because everyone I know is going to die. We are all going to die and it is just a matter of time. All we are doing is changing what we ultimately will die from. The point is, let's be healthy and enjoy and have a nice quality of life while we're living—something we can accomplish by eating real food and healthy food. That's my take-home message for you.

Posted blog: **Mindful Eating**

Mindfulness is the sense of being wholeheartedly present in the moment with whatever is happening then letting go and moving on to the next moment. Mindful eating, then, is learning to be fully engaged with your meals. In short, that means listening to your body and eating as much as it needs. It means eating as much of a variety of foods as recommended here as possible so you get all the micro- and macro-nutrients you need. It means watching your mind as you eat.

Watching your mind as you're eating is the tricky part. Left to its own, the mind will lead us to cravings and overeating, especially of the foods we like. People often mistakenly think that we should focus our attention on enjoying each mouthful "to the fullest." That makes us want more, and wanting more just leads to overeating. Our meals and eating should be nutritious and nourishing, not a source of gluttony.

Like brushing our teeth mindfully, showering mindfully, and urinating mindfully, eating mindfully is a practice we should all do with the intention of mastering it. The *Living in Wellness* mind, after all, is simply learning to be mindful.

Here is an exercise in mindful eating:

Pick a restaurant that you like. Make a reservation there as early as possible for dinner, just when the restaurant opens and when there are the fewest patrons in the restaurant: maybe a Monday night at 5:00 or 6:00 PM. The quieter the restaurant, the fewer distractions there will be to pull you away from your mindfulness. Make the reservation for one. This is an "eat alone" meal.

Arrive a few minutes early. If you are asked where you would like to be seated, say, "Anywhere is all right." When the server arrives and asks if you want a drink, ask for a glass of water without ice. When it's time to order dinner, ask the server to pick an appetizer and an entrée for you. Skip the bread. Mention that you know the restaurant and just want to be surprised. Do mention if you have any allergies.

Mindful eating is about being present with the eating, not about picking and choosing. So far in this exercise, you really haven't picked or chosen much, other than the restaurant.

While you wait for the food, just sit there, still and calm, hands in your lap and allow yourself to sense your body. Let it relax into the seat. Relax your back against the back of the chair. Relax your core into the seat. Next, relax your face, letting go of any tension; then your neck and chest. Finally, settle the soles of your feet comfortably on the floor and relax your hips, thighs and legs.

Focus your mind on your breath. Don't look around for visual stimulation. Don't concern yourself with what others in the restaurant might be doing or eating, or thinking about you. (Believe us, they are all completely self-absorbed in their own food decisions and stress-filled stories; they're not thinking about you.) Don't think about what food might be coming, or when. Just be.

Living in Wellness is about "just being." Just being present with the moment. You can follow your breath, if you want, or just sit peacefully.

When the food arrives, say, "Thank you." Eat slowly. Put your knife and fork down between bites. Fully address your attention to the experience of eating, to what it feels like to press the fork into the food, what it feels like to lift the food to your mouth, how the food feels and tastes in your mouth as you eat it and swallow it. Then let it go and take the next bite. Immediately let go of any judgments about the food.

The point here is to experience the moment, the eating, not to savor or attach to it. Let each moment go so you can greet the next. Mindful eating is about being present with the eating, not about judging, not about liking and disliking. It should be no different from mindfully urinating.

What happens when we eat this way is that we see how our mind drives us to eat more, more, and more. We see how our mind starts us thinking about the next forkful long before we have even swallowed the previous one. We see how hard it is to put down the fork between mouthfuls. We see how we tend to eat those foods on the dish we like best first. We also tend to eat those favorites faster. And we see how hard it is to be with what we are doing.

Living in Wellness asks us to be with what we are doing. To do it appropriately, not greedily. The more appropriate our response, the healthier and more peaceful our life and the lives of those around us will become, including our family and friends, our colleagues and neighbors, and our community.

When you have finished the entrée, the meal's over. Desserts in restaurants are meant to seduce you into eating more than you need. Relax for a few minutes, and thank the server with a minimum of words or mental commentary.

When you leave, just leave, mindfully. That's it. Learn to do this with every meal and you will have conquered your eating issues.

That's mindfulness . . . the source of peace and well-being. And getting to be less fat if that is your goal.

Tips for Mindful Eating At Home

Start the practice of mindful eating with these general guidelines:

1. Don't eat while standing or in front of the refrigerator door.
2. Eat slowly and mindfully. Put your fork down between bites.
3. Skip dessert, unless it's fruit.

Living in Wellness, living with a mindful eye on our body, tells us that being overweight is difficult and can cause health issues. But we recognize that losing weight can also be difficult. So commit, gently but decidedly, to getting to a reasonable weight for you. Check with the doctor with whom you are collaborating to keep you healthy and who will provide guidance to help you reach a more appropriate weight for who you are, for your body. Forget about the "Ideal Body Weight Charts." Eat mindfully, and with patience and, in time, you will be where you need to be. This isn't about how fast you can get there; it is about *Living in Wellness*.

RECIPES

Following are some healthful and delicious recipes from a friend and patient that will show you how easy it is to cook your way to wellness.

Posted blog: **Eat This, and Eat When You're Hungry**

Following is the condensed version of our prescription for healthy eating:

1. *Meat, chicken and fish* — As much as you want to eat, whenever you want to eat, really! This includes beef, pork and ribs, lamb, poultry, eggs (lots of eggs), fish of any type (including herring, sardines, shrimp, crab, lobster, oysters, and shellfish) and cheeses — *in moderation.* Buy pasture-raised, grass-fed animal products and aged cheeses.
2. *"Milks"* — Almond, coconut milk (unsweetened only), or heavy whipping cream.
3. *Fruit* — 1 serving a day...avoid bananas, pineapple or mangos. Focus on berries, apples, oranges and grapefruit.
4. *Water* — filtered, sparkling; unflavored or naturally flavored (add a squeeze of lemon or lime...great) and green tea.
5. *Vegetables* — as much as you like, except potatoes (see following).
6. *Potatoes* — sweet or Yukon gold only and only in moderation, if you must.
7. *Fats* — Butter, cook with it and use it on everything you can. Of course extra virgin olive or coconut oil is good too.
8. *Avocados* — get 'em in you daily.
9. *Homemade mayonnaise* — anytime you want.
10. *Nuts* — raw only, in moderation . . . not peanuts (peanuts are beans, not nuts; even squirrels won't eat them)
11. *Alcohol* — depending on your health and weight-loss goals, for most people, 1 to 2 glasses of wine or beer is ok!

Remember what Hippocrates said: "Let food be your medicine." Eating right is *Living in Wellness*. It is a lot less about pills than about *what* you eat.

Soups

Soup is an ideal vehicle for getting your protein—both vegetable and animal. A big pot of soup can be the start of a family meal or the entree for a satisfying lunch. Many of those included here can be frozen in individual portions then thawed and heated for a quick, "comfort" type dinner after a long, stressful day.

GENTLY CURRIED SWEET POTATO SOUP

Makes 4 to 6 servings

This quick soup has a big, sweet flavor balanced gently with a little curry powder. Serve it in a mug for lunch or as the starter for a family dinner.

4 tablespoons coconut oil
1 medium-sized onion, peeled and chopped
1 tablespoon curry powder
2 cups (16 ounces) mashed sweet potatoes
4 cups chicken stock

Place the coconut oil in a nonstick sauté pan and set over medium heat. Add the onion; mix so that all the onion pieces are lightly coated, and sauté, stirring frequently, until onion becomes translucent, about 6 minutes.

Sprinkle the curry over the onions and cook 2 minutes longer to remove the powdery flavor of the curry. If you're a big curry fan, add an extra tablespoon, or, if you'd prefer, add ½ teaspoon each of ground cumin, ground coriander, and ground cardamom).

Scrape into the bowl of a food processor, add the remaining ingredients, and puree; or combine everything in a large bowl and puree, in batches, in a blender. Heat and serve.

Chili Sweet Potato Soup: Replace the curry with 1 tablespoon chili powder, 1 teaspoon ground cumin, and ½teaspoon crushed dried oregano.

Sweet Potato Bisque: To make bisque in either the recipe or variation above, replace 2 cups of the stock with 2 cups of cream.

EGG DROP SOUP WITH SEAFOOD OR CHICKEN AND CHIVES

Makes 6 servings

This is a simple version of the classic Chinese egg drop soup— but not as thick, with a richer broth flavor and with some fish or chicken added. If there are children, let them watch or help as the egg whites are poured into the spinning soup to form the white threads. In very cold weather, I sometimes stir a little hot Chinese mustard or mushroom soy sauce into the soup just before serving.

4 cups chicken stock
½ tablespoons cornstarch mixed until smooth with 2 tablespoons cold water
3 large eggs beaten with 3 tablespoons cold water
2 cups seafood (leftover diced shrimp or any firm white fish, such as sole, haddock, bass, etc.) or roasted, diced or shredded chicken
2 tablespoons freshly chopped chives

In a large pot, bring the stock to a boil. When the stock boils, stir in the cornstarch and bring back to a boil so the soup will thicken, whisking occasionally. When it has reached a rolling boil, remove the soup from the heat and stir with a large spoon so that the soup is spinning around in a circle. While stirring with one hand to keep the soup moving, slowly pour the egg white mixture, in a very thin stream, into the center of the spinning soup. This will form the traditional threads called "egg drops."

Distribute the seafood or chicken into bowls. Ladle in the soup, sprinkle the top of each with a few chives, and serve.

PARSNIP BISQUE WITH COCONUT

Makes 8 to 10 servings

This soup has a velvety texture and a sweet flavor, with a coconut aroma and a subtle nip of cardamom and ginger.

¼ cup coconut oil
1 small onion, trimmed, coarsely chopped
2 large leeks, white part only, thoroughly washed
1 celery rib, finely chopped
1 pound medium-sized parsnips, washed, trimmed, peeled and cut into 1-inch pieces
5 cups chicken stock
3 cups cream
½ teaspoon ground cardamom
⅛ teaspoon ground ginger
¼ cup unsweetened shredded coconut
A little salt and freshly ground black pepper

Melt the coconut oil in a large soup pot, place over medium heat. Add the onion, leeks, celery and parsnips and sauté until translucent, about 6 minutes, stirring frequently. Add the chicken stock; bring to a boil over high heat. Reduce the heat and simmer for ½ hour. Add the cream and allow to cool.

In small batches, puree the soup in a blender until very smooth, holding the top of the blender securely in place to prevent the soup from erupting all over the kitchen. Strain to remove the bits of coconut, if you want a very smooth soup, then heat and serve.

WILD MUSHROOM SOUP

Makes 8 servings

Laden with strips of wild mushrooms and accented garlic, this soup has an unexpected gentleness.

2 celery ribs, washed and cut into small dices
1 medium size onion, trimmed, peeled, and diced
1 large garlic clove, peeled and very finely chopped
2 pounds shiitake mushrooms, or a mixture of shiitake and other
    wild mushrooms, stems removed, washed and cut into ½-inch
    chunks
7 cups beef broth
1 teaspoon finely chopped fresh thyme
A little salt and freshly ground black pepper

Combine everything except the salt and pepper in a large soup pot. Bring to a boil over high heat, then reduce the heat and simmer for 45 minutes. Season with salt and pepper to taste.

WINTER TOMATO SOUP

Makes 8 servings

By January or February, when it has been months since I have eaten a great, vine-ripened tomato, I make this soup, as a remembrance of summer. This is a simple but interesting, moderately thin soup. The sweet red peppers, rather than competing with the tomatoes, bring out their flavor.

Two 28-ounce cans peeled Italian-style plum tomatoes, undrained
1 tablespoon tomato paste
2 medium-sized sweet red bell peppers, cored and cut into 1-inch
    pieces
2 cups beef broth
1 tablespoon sweet, hot or smoked Hungarian paprika
A little salt
Freshly ground black pepper

In a large soup pot, combine everything except the salt and pepper and bring to a boil over high heat. Reduce the heat and simmer for 30 minutes, stirring occasionally to break up the tomatoes.

In a blender, in small batches, holding the cover securely in place to prevent the soup from spewing all over the kitchen, puree the soup until very smooth.

Return to the soup pot, season with salt and pepper to taste, and reheat before serving.

Leftover soup can be refrigerated for up to 3 days, and frozen for up to 4 months.

THAI-STYLE FISH SOUP WITH LEMONGRASS

Makes 6 servings

This Thai-style soup is made by flavoring a light fish broth with lemongrass and ginger, then straining the broth and adding shrimp, scallops, tomato, and slivers of hot pepper. The seafood adds textural interest to the highly scented soup. The jalapeño pepper can be eliminated if you prefer a milder version.

Lemongrass is a fibrous grass with a straw color that is sold in sticks about two feet long. When cooked, it imparts a sweet, roundly flavored lemon taste, without any of the acidity of lemon juice. It is available in premium supermarkets.

6 small fresh shrimp, peeled, shells reserved

8 cups fish stock (see boxed recipe below)

3 sticks lemongrass, bottoms trimmed; tough, dry outer leaves removed, then cut crosswise (like scallions) with a sturdy serrated knife into ¼-inch pieces

3 quarter-sized disks fresh gingerroot

6 large fresh bay scallops, each carefully cut crosswise into 3 disks

1 small jalapeño pepper, ends trimmed, cut in half lengthwise, seeds removed, and cut into 1/8-inch slivers (the rest of the pepper can he saved for another use)

1 small tomato, cored and cut in half around its middle, then squeezed to remove the seeds, and finally cut into ½-inch dice with a serrated knife

A little salt and freshly ground black pepper

Combine the shrimp shells, stock, lemongrass, and ginger in a large non-aluminum saucepan and bring to a boil over high heat. Lower the heat so the stock is boiling very gently and reduce to 6 cups. Strain through a sieve lined with a dampened towel or cheesecloth and return to the saucepan.

Bring back to a boil; add the shrimp, scallops, the jalapeno slivers, and the diced tomato. Adjust the heat so the stock simmers until the shrimp and scallops have just become opaque, which happens very quickly, about 90 seconds.

Ladle into heated soup bowls or plates. Each should have 3 pieces of scallop, 1 shrimp, and 3 slivers of the pepper. Season with salt and pepper to taste. Serve immediately.

FISH STOCK, BROTH, OR SOUP

Makes 2 quarts

This is a full-flavored fish stock with flavor subtleties from the vegetables, herbs, lemon, and wine. It can be used as a broth or light soup, or as a liquid for poaching fish.

Use the flesh, bones, and tails of white fish such as halibut, grouper, haddock or whitefish. Do not use oily fish such as tuna, swordfish, bluefish, or salmon, as they would give the stock an unpleasant, fishy flavor. Bones can be purchased from the fresh fish section of most premium supermarkets.

With a heavy kitchen knife, cut the tails off the bones, and cut the bones into pieces about 3 inches long, so all the flavor is extracted easily when the stock is simmered. This is a messy procedure, so you might ask the person at the store to do it.

4 pounds fish hones, cut up and thoroughly washed
1 medium-sized onion, trimmed, peeled, and chopped
1 large leek, white part only, split and thoroughly washed
   to remove the grit and chop coarsely
2 celery ribs, washed and thinly sliced or coarsely
   chopped
2 garlic cloves, peeled and coarsely chopped
3 parsley sprigs, washed
1 small lemon, cut into thirds
1 sprig fresh thyme, or ¼ teaspoon dried thyme
1 bay leaf, crumbled
½ teaspoon white peppercorns
1½ cups fine-quality dry white wine
2 quarts cold tap water

Toss all the ingredients into a large non-aluminum pot and bring to a boil over medium heat. Reduce the heat and simmer, partially covered, for 45 minutes.

Carefully ladle the stock into a bowl through a strainer lined with cheesecloth or a dampened, clean kitchen towel, pressing firmly on the bones and vegetables so they release all their liquid. Discard the vegetables and bones.

Fish stock can be refrigerated for 2 or 3 days, or frozen for up to 2 or 3 months.

LOBSTER STEW

Makes 4 servings

This is like an oyster stew, but with lobster instead of the usual oysters. It is simple, expensive, and very impressive, especially considering that it takes less than 10 minutes to make. As there are only 5 ingredients, and virtually no cooking, each ingredient for this elegant soup must be perfect. Use only homemade stocks, very fresh basil leaves, and the freshest lobster meat.

Buy the best fresh lobster meat you can; be certain it is fresh, ask if it has been "previously" frozen. Frozen meat will be tough, dry, and grainy.

1 cup fish stock (see boxed recipe)
1 cup chicken stock (see boxed recipe below)
1 cup cream
12 ounces fresh lobster meat, cut into bite-sized pieces
6 fresh basil leaves, stems removed, then rolled like a cigarette
   and cut crosswise into very thin threads with a very sharp
   chef's knife

In a non-aluminum saucepan, bring the fish stock, chicken stock, and cream to a boil. Add the lobster and basil, reduce the heat, and simmer until the lobster just becomes opaque, about 60 to 90 seconds, no longer. Ladle into soup plates and serve immediately.

Meal-Size Soups

There's something hearty and comforting about having a couple of bowls of soup for dinner with the family and friends especially on rainy or snowy days.

AZTEC CHICKEN SOUP

Makes 10 servings

A hot and cold combination of flavors and textures makes this Aztec-inspired chicken soup refreshing and vibrant. The spicy soup, which includes a variety of vegetables, rice, and chick-peas, is boldly flavored with garlic, spices, and herbs, and is topped, just before serving, with chunks of cold avocado mixed with tomatoes, scallions, and a hot pepper. This is a meal in itself.

12 cups cold water
4 pounds chicken bones, necks, or backs
One 2½ pound chicken, quartered
4 large garlic cloves, peeled and finely chopped
1 tablespoon finely chopped fresh oregano
¼ teaspoon ground cloves
1 tablespoon ground cumin
1 large sprig fresh basil
1 bay leaf, crumbled into 3 or 4 pieces each
1 pound zucchini, washed and sliced ¼ inch thick
1 large green peppers, cored, seeded, and cut into ¼-inch dice
2 celery ribs, washed and sliced ¼ inch thick
1 medium-sized onion, peeled, halved lengthwise, and thinly

For garnish:
1 small avocado, peeled, seeded, and cut into ½-inch dice
2 firm, ripe tomatoes, cored and cut into ¼-inch dice 4 thin scallions, washed and thinly sliced
1 small fresh jalapeño pepper, cored, seeded, and finely chopped
Half a small bunch of cilantro leaves, washed and finely chopped

In a large stock pot, bring the water and the 4 pounds of chicken bones or parts to a boil over medium high heat. Reduce the heat and simmer for 1 hour, partially covered. Strain and return the broth to the pot, skimming off any excess fat on the surface. Add the quartered chicken and simmer for 10 minutes.

In the meantime, combine the garlic, oregano, cloves, cumin, and basil in a food processor and process to form a paste. Stir in the garlic paste and bay leaf and simmer for 45 minutes, partly covered.

Carefully remove the chicken and set aside to cool. Skim the soup again, removing much of the fat and the bay leaf. There should be 10 cups of stock at this point. If not, add water to get that amount. Add the zucchini, green peppers, celery and onion to the soup and simmer until tender, about 15 minutes.

Remove the meat from the chicken, discarding the skin and bones. Using 2 forks, or your fingers, pull the chicken into shreds or pieces small enough to fit onto the spoon when the soup is eaten. Add the chicken to the soup and bring to a boil to reheat the soup.

In a small bowl, mix together the ingredients for the garnish. To serve, ladle into bowls and top generously with the avocado-tomato garnish.

Leftover soup can be stored in the refrigerator for up to 3 days, or frozen for up to 4 months.

PROVENCAL-STYLE FISH SOUP WITH HALIBUT AND FENNEL

Makes 8 servings

This golden soup is textured with tomatoes, and sliced onion, and flavored with chunks of halibut, orange zest, garlic, and parsley. Scented with orange and fennel, it reflects, in an unorthodox way, the kinds of everyday fish soups found in the south of France.

Alternative fish: Any firm white fish can be substituted for the halibut, such as snapper, mahi-mahi, grouper, haddock, or bass.

¼ cup extra virgin olive oil

3 garlic cloves, peeled and very finely chopped

1 large onion, trimmed, peeled, cut in half lengthwise, then thinly sliced

3 strips orange zest, peeled from an orange with a swivel-bladed vegetable peeler, each about 1 inch wide and 3 inches long

2 teaspoons fennel seeds, tied in cheesecloth

2 small tomatoes, cored and cut in half around the middle, then squeezed to remove the seeds and cut into ½ inch dice

1 quart fish stock (see boxed recipe above)

¼ teaspoon crushed saffron threads

1 pound fresh halibut fillets, cut into ½-inch cubes

2½ to 3 pounds firm-fleshed white fish (see note above), cut into 1-inch chunks

A little salt and freshly ground black pepper

3 tablespoons finely chopped fresh parsley

For garnish:
Rouille (see boxed recipe below)

Place a large nonstick sauté pan over medium heat. When hot, add the olive oil, then the garlic and onion. Stir until all the vegetables are coated with the oil. Cook for 6 minutes, reducing the heat to prevent browning, and stirring frequently, until the onion is tender and translucent. Scrape into a non-aluminum soup pot.

Add the orange zest, fennel seed, tomatoes, fish stock, and saffron. Bring to a boil over high heat, then reduce the heat and simmer for 20 minutes, stirring occasionally.

Add the fish and simmer until fish is just tender, about 3 minutes. Taste and add a little salt, if necessary, and some pepper.

Ladle into soup bowls and sprinkle each with about a teaspoon of the chopped parsley. Serve immediately, passing the rouille so that each guest can add as much as they want.

Rouille

> 6 large garlic cloves, peeled and roughly chopped
> 1 or 2 very small, fresh, hot red peppers (such as Serranos), split and seeded
> 2 tablespoons tomato paste
> 3 tablespoons olive oil
> Juice of ½ lemon
> 1 teaspoon hot Hungarian paprika
> ¼ teaspoon salt
> ½ teaspoon freshly ground black pepper
> ½ cup fish or chicken stock (see boxed recipes)

Puree everything in a food processor until very smooth. Taste carefully; it may need a little more salt.

---

1. Your diet should be high in fat, moderate in animal protein and low to moderate in carbohydrates.
2. Calorie counting is not encouraged, neither is portion control.
3. Eat unlimited amounts of saturated fats like coconut oil and butter or clarified butter. Beef tallow, lard and duck fat are also good, but only if they come from healthy and well-treated animals. Beef or lamb tallow is a better choice than lamb or duck fat. Olive, avocado and macadamia oil are also good fats to use in salads and to drizzle over food, but not for cooking. Cook with butter and pure (virgin) coconut oil.
4. Eat generous amounts of animal protein. This includes red meat, poultry, pork, eggs, organs (liver, kidney, heart, other) wild-caught fish and shellfish. Don't be afraid to eat the fatty cuts; all meals with proteins should contain fat as well. Learn to cook with stocks and broths that you make from animal bones.
5. Eat good amounts of fresh or frozen vegetables either cooked or raw and served with fat. Starchy vegetables such as sweet potatoes and yams are also great as a source of non-toxic carbohydrates.
6. Eat low to moderate amounts of fruits and nuts. Try to eat mostly fruits low in sugar (the occasional banana) and high in antioxidants like berries. If you have an autoimmune disease, have a digestive problem or are trying to lose weight faster, consider eliminating fruits and nuts altogether.
7. Preferably choose pasture-raised and grass-fed meat. If not possible, choose lean cuts of meat and supplement your fat with coconut oil, butter or clarified butter. Also when possible choose organic, local and seasonal fruits and vegetables.
8. Cut from your diet all cereal grains and legumes. This includes, but is not limited to, wheat, rye, barley, oats, corn, brown rice, soy, peanuts, kidney beans, pinto beans, navy beans and black eyed peas.

9. Cut out all vegetable, hydrogenated and partially hydrogenated oils including, but not limited to, margarine, soybean oil, corn oil, Crisco, peanut oil, canola oil, safflower oil and sunflower oil. Olive oil and avocado oil are fine, but don't cook with them; use them in salad dressings and to drizzle over prepared food. Cook with butter and coconut oil.
10. Eliminate sugar, soft drinks, all packaged products and juices (including fruit juices).
11. Eliminate dairy products other than butter and maybe heavy cream. You don't need dairy.
12. Eat when you're hungry and don't stress if you skip a meal or even two. You don't have to eat three square meals a day; do what feels most natural.

A BIG BOILED DINNER FOR A FAMILY OR PARTY MEAL

Makes 8 or more servings

Most cuisines have a soup like this that simply outgrew its pot. In Italy, it's a bollito misto; in France, a pot-au-feu; in this country, a New England boiled dinner. This recipe leans toward the Italian version, although no tortellini is added to the soup. It is a formal, deep-winter meal that generates a broth as the first course, and slices of beef and chicken and an assortment of vegetables as the entree.

Serve with a selection of mustards (coarsely textured mustard, a smooth Dijon-style or Dusseldorf mustard, a Creole mustard, or a flavored mustard) and cornichons (tiny, tart pickles from France). This soup can be made a day or two ahead.

For the broth:
8 cups (2 quarts) chicken or vegetable stock
3 carrots, scrubbed, trimmed, and cut into 3 or 4 pieces each
2 celery ribs, washed and cut into 3 or 4 pieces each
2 large onions, ends trimmed, peeled, and quartered
3 garlic cloves, unpeeled
A 2-inch chunk of fresh gingerroot, unpeeled
2 bay leaves, crumbled
2 teaspoons dried thyme
1 teaspoon dried rosemary
½ teaspoon dried oregano

The meats:
A 2-pound rump roast or bottom round, trimmed of some of its
    excess fat
A 3-pound chicken, excess fat pulled from the vent end, and trussed

The vegetables:
4 cups (1 quart) chicken or vegetable broth (boxed recipes below)
16 pearl onions, trimmed and peeled
2 medium-sized turnips, thickly peeled and cut into 6 wedges each

8 medium-sized leeks, white parts only, thoroughly washed (the
ends can be split, if necessary, to rinse out the grit, but the leeks
should be kept whole for serving)

2 fresh fennel bulbs, tops and cores removed, cut into quarters,
sixths or eighths, depending on the size (enough to make 2 or
3 wedges for each person)

2 medium-sized carrots, trimmed, scrubbed, and cut into 1½-inch
lengths

In a very large soup kettle or stockpot, combine all the ingredients
for the broth. Bring to a boil; then add the beef. Adjust the heat so the
liquid simmers, and cook for 3 hours. The beef should feel tender when
pierced with a carving fork.

While the beef is simmering, fill a large saucepan with the additional
quart of broth. Bring to a boil, and then add the vegetables, one at a
time. Cook until tender, then remove, cool under running cold water,
and set aside. Bring the broth back to a boil before adding the next
vegetable. If preparing this several hours or even a day ahead, moisten
the vegetables after they have been cooked and cooled with a little
broth from the pot, cover tightly, and refrigerate.

After 3 hours, carefully slip the chicken into the simmering liquid
in the stockpot, arranging it atop or next to the beef. There should be
enough liquid to cover the chicken; if not, add more chicken stock or
water. Simmer for 45 to 60 minutes longer to cook the chicken and
finish cooking the beef.

Remove the beef and chicken to a platter and set aside. If preparing
this meal several hours or even a day ahead, place the meats in a
shallow dish, cover with plastic wrap, and refrigerate.

Strain the meat broth, discarding the vegetables that have been
cooked for the last 4 hours. Remove all the fat from the top of the broth.
Cool, then cover and refrigerate the broth if this meal is being made
ahead.

About half an hour before serving (an hour if everything has been
refrigerated), pour the broth back into the pot, bring to a boil over high
heat, add the beef and chicken and all the vegetables, and adjust
the heat so the broth simmers. Simmer for 20 to 30 minutes, until
everything is very hot, then turn off the heat.

To begin the meal, carefully ladle a cup of the broth into hot soup plates and serve. Next, arrange the meats on a carving board, and the vegetables in a variety of large, attractive serving bowls.

Carve the meats at the table, arranging a slice or two of the beef and a slice or two of the chicken on each plate, then surround with 2 or 3 pieces of each of the vegetables. Pass mustards and cornichons separately.

CHICKEN STOCK, BROTH, OR SOUP

Makes 4 quarts

Although there are technical differences between a stock, a broth, and a soup—the stock is the weakest, the broth moderately flavored, and the soup well flavored—for home cooking those distinctions have essentially disappeared. Today, the words are used interchangeably to indicate a full-flavored liquid.

Using a generous amount of chicken, especially the bony parts, like necks, backs, and wings, with some vegetables added to balance the flavor, makes the best-flavored broth. The secret to making a great stock is to simmer it for many hours. Three to 4 hours will make a good stock; 5 hours a fine broth; and 6 hours a great broth. These can be frozen for up to 3 months.

About 8 pounds of chicken and bones (ideally a 4- to 5-pound roasting chicken and 3 or 4 pounds of necks, backs, and wings can be used, although 2 large roasters, cut into serving-size pieces, or all chicken bones will do)

6 quarts cold tap water
4 celery ribs, washed and cut into 2- to 3-inch lengths
4 medium-sized carrots, trimmed, scrubbed, and cut into
    2- to 3-inch lengths
3 medium-sized onions, trimmed, peeled, and quartered
1 large turnip, thickly peeled and quartered

3 large leeks, white parts only, slit, washed thoroughly
   to remove the grit, and cut into 2-inch chunks
2 large tomatoes, cored and cut in half
3 garlic cloves, peeled
2 teaspoons dried thyme
1 teaspoon dried rosemary
4 or 5 parsley sprigs
1 teaspoon black peppercorns
4 whole cloves
3 crumbled bay leaves

In a very large soup kettle or stockpot, combine all the ingredients. There should be enough water to cover everything by at least an inch. If not, add more water. Bring to a boil over medium heat, then reduce the heat and simmer, partially covered, for 4 to 6 hours. Occasionally, skim the stock to remove the fat, foam, and sediment that have risen to the surface.

When the stock has simmered for 1 or 2 hours and the meat is tender, remove the meaty pieces (such as the breast and thighs), cut the meat off the bones, and reserve for a recipe calling for cooked chicken. Return the bones and skin to the pot and continue cooking.

Carefully ladle the stock through a strainer lined with cheesecloth or a dampened, clean kitchen towel. Discard the vegetables and bones.

Refrigerate the stock, then remove the fat that has congealed on the surface.

BROWN BEEF STOCK, OR BROTH, OR SOUP

Makes 4 quarts

Most home cooks rarely make beef stock, which requires browning the beef, bones, and vegetables in the oven, deglazing the roasting pan, and cooking for 24 hours. Unfortunately, there really is no good alternative homemade beef stock. Canned beef stock is a poor substitute, and rehydrated bouillon cubes are worse.

Begin the stock early in the morning. Just before bed, divide it into several bowls, cover, and refrigerate. In the morning, combine everything again, bring to a boil over high heat, reduce the heat, and continue simmering until done.

The beef bones and knuckles for this recipe need to be cut into pieces with a saw. Some supermarket butchers are cooperative enough to do this, as it cannot be done at home; a local butcher will almost always be willing to cut up bones for you.

Like chicken stock, beef stock can be frozen for up to 3 months.

4 pounds beef chuck, trimmed of fat and cut into 4 or 5 pieces
3 pounds beef bones, sawed into 1-inch pieces
2 to 3 pounds veal knuckle bones, sawed into 1-inch pieces
2 medium-sized onions, trimmed, peeled, and halved
3 celery stalks, washed and cut into 3 or 4 pieces each
3 carrots, trimmed, scrubbed, and cut into 3 or 4 pieces each
3 large leeks, white parts only, ends split and washed thoroughly to remove all grit, but left whole
6 garlic cloves, unpeeled
1 quart hottest possible tap water
5 quarts cold tap water
1 teaspoon dried thyme

2 teaspoons dried rosemary
4 whole cloves
4 bay leaves, crumbled

Preheat the oven to 375 degrees F.

Evenly scatter the chuck, beef bones, veal knuckle, onions, celery, carrots, leeks, and garlic in a single layer in a large roasting pan. Roast until the meat, bones, and vegetables are well browned but not burned, about 11/2 hours, turning them 2 or 3 times during the roasting so they color evenly. It is essential that the bones do not burn. With a large spoon and tongs, carefully transfer the meat, bones, and vegetables to a very large stockpot.

Pour the fat out of the roasting pan and place the pan across 2 burners set on high heat. Add the quart of hot water to the pan, and scrape the bottom of the pan so that all the brown, encrusted bits mix into the water as it comes to a boil. Carefully pour into the stockpot with the beef, bones, and vegetables.

Add the cold water, thyme, rosemary, cloves, and bay leaves to the stockpot and bring to a boil over medium high heat. Reduce the heat and simmer, partially covered, for 24 hours. Occasionally, skim the stock to remove the fat, foam, and sediment that have risen to the surface.

Carefully ladle the stock into a large bowl through a strainer lined with cheesecloth or a dampened, clean kitchen towel.

Refrigerate the stock, then remove the fat that has congealed on the surface.

Dips and Spreads

Intensely flavored dips, rather than just being an accent on the edge of an overly salted, greasy chip or cracker, can be a culinary center of attention when served over or with eggs, burgers, and roasts, or with raw or cooked vegetables. All of the dips in this section can be prepared 2 or 3 days ahead. Store them in a covered container in the refrigerator, and stir just before serving.

MIXED HERB, CAPER AND ANCHOVY DIP

Makes about 2 cups

This dip abounds with the flavors often found in Italian green sauces, and like those sauces, it is especially tasty on poached fish or chicken.

2 cups real mayonnaise, not the shelf-stable type in a jar
2 tablespoons Dijon mustard
¼ cup capers, rinsed well under running cold water
2 garlic cloves, peeled
6 anchovy fillets, rinsed well under running cold water
¼ cup coarsely chopped fresh basil
½ cup coarsely chopped fresh parsley
¼ cup coarsely chopped fresh dill
½ cup coarsely chopped chives
¼ cup extra virgin olive oil
Juice of 1 small lemon
Freshly ground black pepper

In a food processor, combine the mayonnaise with the mustard, capers, garlic, anchovies, basil, parsley, dill, chives, olive oil and lemon juice. Process, pulsing frequently, until everything is very finely chopped. Season with pepper. Refrigerate in a covered container until needed.

SUN-DRIED TOMATO AND DILL DIP

Makes about 3 cups

This is a thick dip, richly flavored with sun-dried tomatoes and accented with fresh dill. To make a spicier dip, add 1 teaspoon chili powder, 1 teaspoon hot or sweet Hungarian paprika, and ½ teaspoon crushed dried oregano to the food processor with the other ingredients.

2 cups plain, full-fat unflavored Greek yogurt
1 cup sun-dried tomatoes
½cup coarsely chopped fresh curly parsley
¼ cup chopped fresh tarragon
1 garlic clove, peeled
¼ cup extra virgin olive oil
A little salt and freshly ground black pepper

In a food processor, combine all the ingredients except the salt and pepper and pulse frequently until the tomatoes have been finely chopped and the dip is mostly smooth, although speckled, with finely chopped dill. Taste and season with salt and pepper.

EASY PROCESSOR HOMEMADE MAYONNAISE

4 large pasture-raised fresh large egg yolks
1/2 teaspoon salt
1/4 teaspoon freshly ground black pepper
1 teaspoon Dijon mustard
Juice of half a lemon or 1 tablespoon white balsamic
    vinegar
3/4 cup extra virgin olive oil

With the metal chopping blade in place, add the yolks, salt, pepper, mustard, and lemon juice or vinegar and process for 30 seconds.

Continue processing, very very slowly drizzling a quarter cup of the oil through the feed tube about a teaspoon at a time. Let each teaspoon incorporate fully before adding the next, otherwise the mayonnaise will curdle. Process for another 15 or 20 seconds, then slowly add the remaining oil, a tablespoon or two at a time, allowing it to emulsify after each addition before adding more oil.

Taste and adjust the seasoning; add a tablespoon or two of cold water if the mayonnaise is thicker than you'd like.

EGGPLANT DIP

Makes about 3 cups

This light dip can be used as a spread or sauce, either cold or at room temperature. In winter, when I originally developed this recipe, I substituted sweet red bell peppers for the tomatoes. Sometimes I eliminate the hot pepper.

One 2-pound eggplant, stem trimmed, cut in half lengthwise
2 to 3 tablespoons olive oil
2 large tomatoes, washed, cored, seeded, and cut into ¼-inch dice
½ small jalapeno, trimmed, halved, seeded, and finely chopped
2 scallions, finely chopped
3 tablespoons olive oil
1 small bunch cilantro, washed and finely chopped
Juice of 1 lime
Freshly ground black pepper

Place the eggplant, cut side down, on a baking sheet that has been generously rubbed with olive oil and bake in a 350-degree oven until tender when pierced deeply with a toothpick, about 45 minutes. In the meantime, mix together in a large bowl the tomato, hot pepper, scallions, oil, cilantro and lime juice.

When eggplant is cooked, using a large spoon scrape out the flesh onto a cutting board and chop into fine pieces. Discard the skin. Stir into the tomato and scallion mixture, taste; adjust the flavors, adding more cilantro or lime juice if needed to make the taste bouncy and alive, and season generously with pepper.

Vegetables

Loading up on veggies satisfies and fills you. Keep in mind that all vegetables suit our diet with the exception of white potatoes.

STEAMED ASPARAGUS WITH SUN-DRIED TOMATO SAUCE

Makes 4 servings

This is a sprightly and dramatic-looking appetizer for a cool spring day; a simple, light, sensual combination of tastes and textures. Sun-dried California tomatoes, with their slightly acidic flavor and rich, natural sweetness, are softened in some broth and quickly made into a thick chutney-like sauce that is spooned over fresh asparagus. You can substitute broccoli florets for the asparagus spears.

> 1 pound asparagus, washed and lower halves peeled if stalks are thick and woody
> Sun-dried Tomato Sauce (recipe follows)

Place 2 inches of water in the bottom of a steamer, insert the steaming basket, cover, and bring to a boil. When the steamer is filled with steam, add the asparagus, cover, reduce the heat to medium, and steam until just tender, about 5 to 6 minutes.

Stack the asparagus neatly on serving plates and spoon the warm sauce over them. Serve immediately.

SUNDRIED TOMATO SAUCE

Makes about 2 cups

This sauce is lusciously bold in flavor. It's great on burgers or served with roasted beef or lamb.

1 cup sun-dried tomatoes, if packed in oil, drain thoroughly
½ cup olive oil
2 tablespoons balsamic or sherry vinegar
2 tablespoons finely chopped fresh basil or cilantro
Freshly ground black pepper to taste

In a food processor, puree all the ingredients to form a thick, almost smooth sauce.

BROCCOLI WITH ONIONS

Makes 4 servings

Broccoli florets enmeshed in tender strands of sweet onion and flavored with fresh herbs make a simple, pure dish, far better tasting than its humble ingredients would indicate.

¼ cup unsalted butter
2 medium onions, peeled, cut in half lengthwise,
    then very thinly sliced
1 garlic clove, peeled and finely chopped
1 bunch broccoli, cut into florets
3 tablespoons finely chopped fresh parsley, basil, or cilantro
Salt and freshly ground black pepper

Melt the butter in a large nonstick skillet over medium heat. Add the onions and garlic and toss until lightly coated. Cook over medium low heat, stirring frequently, until very limp and lightly browned, about 15 to 20 minutes.

Meanwhile, cook the broccoli in boiling water until tender, about 8 to 10 minutes. Drain and cool under running cold tap water to set the color and stop the cooking. Drain thoroughly and pat dry.

Mix the broccoli into the onions, increase the heat to moderate, and toss until very hot. Add the herbs and black pepper, mix well and serve immediately.

BRUSSELS SPROUTS WITH NUTMEG

Makes 4 servings

Small, young Brussels sprouts have a sweet, fragrant, slightly *nutlike character. Older sprouts develop a strong cabbage flavor and "off" odor. Choose the youngest, smallest sprouts available.*

Whole nutmegs, shaped like an inch-long football, are available *in the spice section of many premium supermarkets, and in health food stores. You can usually find an inexpensive aluminum grater. Freshly grated nutmeg has a sweet, nutty fragrance, unlike the powdery, lackluster ground nutmeg in spice-rack jars.*

    4 cups chicken stock
    1 pound fresh young Brussels sprouts, any damaged outer leaves
        removed, bottoms trimmed
    3 Tablespoons olive oil
    A little salt and freshly grated nutmeg

In a medium-sized saucepan, bring the stock to a boil over high heat. There should be enough stock to cover the sprouts when they are added. Add the sprouts, and when the stock returns to a boil, reduce the heat and simmer until the sprouts are just tender, about 6 minutes.

Immediately drain, toss with the olive oil so the sprouts begin to glisten, then season lightly with salt and grate a little nutmeg over the sprouts, just enough to give them a fragrance of nutmeg. Do not over flavor them, or the nutmeg will hide the sweetness of the vegetable.

GREEN BEANS WITH CHERMOULA SAUCE

Makes 6 servings

Tender, small pieces of fresh green beans are gently coated here with chermoula, the lemony, mildly spicy sauce from North Africa. The balance of flavors is sprightly and will add a sparkle to almost any meal.

1½ pounds green beans, ends trimmed and strung if necessary,
    then cut into 1-inch pieces
Chermoula sauce (recipe follows)

Fill a large saucepan with water and bring to a boil over high heat. Add the green beans, reduce the heat to medium, and boil until beans are quite tender, about 10 to 12 minutes.

Drain thoroughly, then toss with enough chermoula (about 1/3 cup) so all the beans are coated. Serve immediately.

CHERMOULA SAUCE

Makes about 1 cup

This is the North African version of Mexico's salsa — hot, sometimes fiery; balanced, acidic, and bold. Drizzle on vegetables, hot or cold, or use to accompany roast, steaks or chops. It's especially good with chicken.

1 small bunch cilantro
½ bunch fresh curly parsley
3 garlic cloves, peeled
Juice of 1 large lemon
Juice of 2 small limes
1 tablespoon tomato paste
½ teaspoon salt
½ teaspoon freshly ground black pepper
2 tablespoons hot Hungarian paprika
1½ teaspoons ground cumin
¼ teaspoon cayenne, or more or none, depending on how hot you
    want the sauce

Combine all the ingredients in a food processor and process until the herbs are very finely chopped and a thick, well-blended sauce forms.

Chermoula can be stored in a tightly covered jar for up to 4 days in the refrigerator.

GREEN BEANS AND FENNEL

Makes 4 servings

Green beans and fennel, both cut the same size and cooked until tender, are a natural pair, enhancing each other's sweetness. The light cream-and-dill dressing binds them, enhancing the mild anise flavor of the fennel and relating it to the beans.

12 ounces green beans, washed, ends snapped off and cut into 1-inch lengths
2 large fennel bulbs, stalks trimmed, discolored outer layers discarded, and inner layers cut into 1/3-inch-wide strips, then cut into 1-inch lengths (the fennel pieces should be about the same size as the cut beans)
2 tablespoons finely chopped fresh dill
¼ cup full-fat sour cream
A little salt and freshly ground black pepper

Bring a large saucepan of water to a boil over high heat. Add the beans and cook until tender and not at all crisp, about 9 minutes. Immediately drain and cool under running cold water. Drain and set aside. Cook the fennel in the same manner until tender, about 7 minutes.

When fennel is tender, add the cooked beans to the pot with the fennel and cook just long enough for the beans to heat. Drain well, toss with the dill and sour cream and serve.

CURRIED CAULIFLOWER

Makes 6 servings

Curried cauliflower, with its bright yellow color and mild-tasting spiciness, is an excellent accompaniment to chicken, game and lamb.

3 tablespoons olive oil
1 large onion, peeled and finely chopped
A 1-inch piece fresh gingerroot, peeled and finely chopped
1 large garlic clove, peeled and finely chopped
Juice of ½ large lemon
¼ cup chicken stock
2 tablespoons curry powder
½ teaspoon ground cumin
½ teaspoon ground coriander
¼ teaspoon ground cardamom
1 medium-sized head cauliflower, cored and cut into small florets

Place a large sauté pan over medium heat. When hot, add the oil, onion, ginger and garlic and toss until everything is coated with oil. Reduce the heat to medium low and cook, stirring frequently, for 10 minutes without browning the onion.

In a small bowl, stir together the lemon juice, stock, curry powder, cumin, coriander, and cardamom. Pour into the sauté pan and swirl around to mix well. Add the cauliflower and toss until evenly colored. Reduce the heat to low, cover, and cook until cauliflower is tender, about 6 to 8 minutes, shaking the pan or stirring once or twice. Serve immediately.

SPRING DANDELION GREENS WITH MUSHROOMS

Makes 4 servings

Tender young dandelion greens, sometimes called spring dandelion greens, need considerably less cooking time than older greens, and are intense but not overly. Here they are gently stewed with mushrooms and flavored with a little garlic and ginger.

1 very large onion, peeled, and chopped
2 garlic cloves, peeled and chopped
A 1-inch chunk fresh gingerroot, peeled and very finely chopped
¼ cup olive oil
8 ounces baby Portobello mushrooms, washed and quartered
16 ounces spring dandelion greens, thoroughly washed and thick
    stems cut off, then gathered together tightly and cut into ½-inch
    shreds
A little salt and freshly ground black pepper

Place a very large pot over medium low heat. Add the olive oil, onions, garlic and ginger and cook, stirring occasionally, until the onions are translucent, about 6 minutes. Add the mushrooms and greens, mix well, cover loosely, and cook until greens are just tender, about 15 minutes. Season with salt and pepper to taste.

STEWED OKRA AND TOMATOES WITH CILANTRO

Makes 6 servings

Properly cooked, okra has a fresh, sensual texture and is one of the great joys of the summer garden. Here, it is stewed with lots of onions and tomatoes and flavored with cilantro, ginger, lime juice and a few shreds of jalapeno. The combination bursts with energy.

Buy fresh, young okra no more than about 2 inches in length, and when trimming, cut off the stem without exposing the soft inside to ensure the okra is tender. Longer, older, often brown-gray blotched okra can be both tough and slimy.

4 tablespoons butter
3 garlic cloves, peeled and chopped
½ small jalapeño pepper, trimmed, seeded, and cut into the thinnest possible threads (optional)
A ¾-inch piece fresh gingerroot, peeled and very finely chopped
1 medium-sized onion, peeled and finely chopped 1½ pounds fresh okra, stem ends trimmed
One 28-ounce can crushed tomatoes in puree
Juice of 1 lime
1 small hunch cilantro, coarsely chopped
A little freshly ground black pepper

Place a large saucepan or small pot over medium-low heat melt the butter, then add the garlic, jalapeño, ginger, and onion and toss. Cook for 6-8 minutes, stirring frequently and reducing the heat if necessary to prevent browning.

Add the okra, tomatoes and lime juice, mix well, and bring to a boil over medium high heat, stirring occasionally to prevent scorching. Reduce the heat and simmer, partially covered, until okra is tender, about 25 minutes, stirring occasionally.

Stir in the cilantro and season very lightly with pepper. Serve in bowls.

SWEET RED PEPPER RAGOUT

Makes 6 servings

Hungarian paprika adds a shadow of warmth to this richly textured, sweet pepper stew, with lemon juice balancing the flavors. The peppers become very soft as they stew, but retain their fire-engine red color.

You can change this ragout into a spread simply by cutting the peppers in ½-inch dice instead of strips. The spread can be spooned onto chicken or fish. For an interesting variation, use yellow or orange peppers (with curry powder instead of paprika).

2 garlic cloves, peeled and finely chopped
1 large red onion, peeled and thinly sliced
3 tablespoons olive oil
1 tablespoon sweet Hungarian paprika
3 pounds large sweet red bell peppers, washed, cored, and cut into
    1/4-inch strips
Juice of 1 lemon
A little salt and freshly ground black pepper

Combine the garlic, onions and olive oil in a large, heavy pot set over medium heat. Cook until wilted, about 5 minutes, stirring once or twice.

Add the paprika and mix well (the onions will become tangled). Cover and cook for 1 minute.

Add the peppers and lemon juice, stir to break up the clumps of onion, cover, and cook until tender and wilted down to about half the original volume, 15 to 20 minutes, stirring occasionally.

Cook, uncovered, stirring occasionally, until most of the liquid has evaporated, about 15 minutes. Season with salt and pepper.

EMERALD SPINACH WITH HIDDEN HERBS

Makes 4 servings

This exceptionally delicious spinach recipe sparkles with flavor, the hidden herbs adding an unexpected depth to the brilliant green leaves.

- 3 tablespoons unsalted butter
- 1 pound fresh spinach, thick stems removed, thoroughly washed, drained, and coarsely chopped
- 2 bunches fresh coriander, rinsed under running cold water, stems removed
- Salt and freshly ground black pepper

Melt the butter in a large pot set over medium high heat, then add the spinach and stir frequently until just wilted, about 5 minutes. Meanwhile, coarsely chop enough of the coriander and stir into the spinach. Season with salt and pepper. Serve immediately.

JULIENNED SUMMER SQUASH SKINS

Makes 6 servings

This recipe uses just the skin, which has most of the flavor and nutrients, of yellow and green zucchini.

3 pounds yellow crookneck summer squash (preferably about 2 inches in diameter), washed, ends trimmed, and cut into 3-inch lengths
2 pounds zucchini (preferably about 2 inches in diameter), washed, ends trimmed, and cut into 3-inch lengths
1 tablespoon very finely chopped fresh chives
2 tablespoons unsalted butter
A little salt and freshly ground black pepper

Using a mandolin or plastic vegetable cutter, julienne just the squash skins, reserving the flesh for another use, if you wish. Bring a large pot of water to a rapid boil. Drop all the julienned skins into the water at once, stir and cook until just about tender, about 1 to 2 minutes. Drain immediately, toss gently with the chives and butter, and season with a little salt and very little pepper. Serve immediately.

RUSSIAN SUMMER VEGETABLE SALAD

Makes 6 to 8 servings

With vegetables fresh from the garden, the farm or the farmers' market, this is one of the most refreshing ways to celebrate summer. Although I usually find I have nibbled my way through a third of this salad before it gets into the refrigerator, it should be served cold.

Texturally, the salad is best when all the vegetables are cut to the same size, about ½-inch dice. For a more subtle flavor, cut the vegetables into ¼-inch dice. For a rustic feel, chop them coarsely and unevenly.

4 large vine-ripened tomatoes, washed, cored, seeded and diced
4 medium-sized pickling (Kirby) cucumbers, scrubbed and diced, or
    1 large cucumber, peeled, seeded and diced
1 each sweet red, yellow and orange bell peppers, washed, cored,
    seeded and diced
1 large bunch fresh dill, washed, shaken dry, and finely chopped
    (about 1 cup)
About 1 cup full-fat sour cream
A little salt and freshly ground black pepper

In a large bowl, mix everything together and toss gently. Taste and season with salt and pepper.

Refrigerate the salad for an hour or two before serving, to allow the flavors to mellow.

Fish

With the high amount of oils that fish contain, these are ideal staples of the lifestyle program guidelines to healthy eating.

SPICY SALMON FILLETS

Makes 6 servings

These succulent, moist, perfectly cooked salmon fillets are coated with chili powder to bring out their rich character.

½ cup hot or sweet chili powder
¼ teaspoon salt
3 tablespoons olive oil
A 2-pound skinless fresh salmon fillet, cut into 4 equal pieces

Preheat the oven to 450 degrees F.

Pour the chili powder and salt into a bowl and mix with the oil. Add the salmon pieces, one at a time, rolling the fillets in the spice mixture and pressing gently on the fish so that the fillets are evenly coated on all sides.

Arrange the salmon in a large baking dish so that none of the pieces are touching. Bake uncovered for 10 minutes.

Serve immediately; or, to serve cold, transfer to a cold plate or dish, cover, and refrigerate until needed.

SEARED HALIBUT

Makes 6 servings

When fish is seared, it develops a crust with a deep mahogany color. The crust not only seals in the natural flavors and juices, making the fish tender and moist, but adds sweetness as well.

Firm white fish, like halibut, grouper, mahi-mahi and red snapper, with their mild flavor, sear exceptionally well. Here, halibut is seared and served with spicy North African sauce. In the variations following, salmon and tilefish are seared and served with different sauces.

1 pound fresh halibut in a 1-inch thick fillet, quartered
2 tablespoons extra virgin olive oil
1 recipe *Chermoula Sauce* (see recipe above)

Pat the halibut very dry so it will sear well.

Place a large nonstick sauté pan over medium heat. When it is hot, add the oil. Add the halibut and reduce the heat to medium low. Cook until golden brown on the bottom, 3 or 4 minutes, without moving the fish. The halibut should be a deep golden mahogany color, but not blackened or burned. Adjust the heat, if necessary, to achieve this color in the time specified. Carefully turn the fish and cook the other side until golden, about 4 more minutes.

While the halibut is cooking, warm the sauce, either in a microwave oven or in a saucepan on the stovetop. Spoon chermoula onto plates and top with the seared halibut. Serve immediately.

Eggs

This segment isn't a primer on eggs, even though eggs should be an everyday staple of your healthy eating. Instead, it consists of just two unique recipes for using eggs that are particularly versatile and healthy: egg wraps. The recipes use eggs to encase stuffings and fillings that are healthy and infinitely variable. The fillings can make them into a simple everyday dish or a rich and unusual company fare.

FRITTATAS

These are great for breakfast, brunch, snacks. Anytime, really. A frittata is a big golden brown omelet that is baked, rather than sautéed. It is easy to make, can be kept in the refrigerator for several days, and looks really impressive. It is an easy way to use up leftover meat or fish and vegetables.

Serve with bacon or sausage for breakfast or brunch, with a salad for lunch, wrap chunks in sliced prosciutto to use as an appetizer, accompany it with slaw at a picnic or top with garnishes like avocados, fresh tomatoes, fresh chopped herbs, even a tapenade or pesto. As with burgers, have fun with the toppings.

Here's how it works: you fill a 9- to 10-inch non-stick sauté pan with 3-4 cups full of diced-up cooked stuff (such as meats or chicken or fish, vegetables and cheese: great tasting stuff in any combination you like), then you pour a dozen eggs over it all and bake it in the oven for 40 minutes. The result is a spectacular, puffy, golden brown omelet that you invert onto a plate and serve, either straight from the over or later, cooled to room temperature. Leftovers can be kept in the refrigerator, then quickly warmed in the microwave.

2 tablespoons olive oil
4-6 cups *stuff* as filling (see below)
12 eggs
¼ cup water
Salt and freshly ground black pepper

Heat the oven to 350°F.

Rub a 9- to 10-inch sauté pan with the olive oil. Add the stuff to the pan, distributing it evenly. Beat the eggs and water with a whisk until welled combined and all the yolks and whites are blended; whisk in salt and pepper to taste, then pour evenly across the top of the filling so that the egg fills the pan.

Bake for 40 minutes. The frittata should be puffed and golden brown. Test for doneness by inserting the tip of a small sharp knife into the center of the frittata. If it comes out clean, it's done. If not, cook for another 5 to 6 minutes and test again.

When done, carefully place a plate over the top of the pan and flip. The frittata will drop right onto the plate, ready for serving.

Stuff for fillings:

Easy Breakfast Frittata – Use two cups of diced cooked breakfast sausage and 1 cup diced cheddar.

Ham and Cheese Frittata – This can be a simple everyday ham and cheese (using boiled ham and processed Swiss) or an elegant ham and Swiss using Serrano Ham or Prosciutto and an aged French gruyere. In either case use 1½ cups of each. The everyday version almost screams for some mustard, the more sophisticated version could be drizzled with some truffle oil or a boldly flavored extra virgin olive oil.

Mushroom and Fontina Frittata with Chicken – Use 1 cup sautéed mushrooms, any combination of mushrooms you want, with 2 cups leftover diced chicken, 1 cup shredded Fontina cheese and ½ cup coarsely chopped fresh parsley. Serve with basil pesto or one of the dips (see recipes).

Salmon, Asparagus and Caramelized Onion Frittata – Use a cup-and-a-half or two cups of cooked fresh salmon, and a cup of cooked fresh asparagus that have been cut into 1-inch pieces, and a cup or so of caramelized onions. Serve with sour cream sprinkled with fresh chopped dill.

Chorizo, Cheddar and Spinach Frittata – Use 1 pound cooked, diced chorizo, ½ pound diced cheddar, ½ pound cooked spinach and a large bunch of fresh cilantro coarsely chopped. Serve with salsa verde and sour cream, if you want.

Sweet or Hot Italian Sausage, Mozzarella, and Sundried Tomatoes – Use 1 pound cooked sausage(sliced or diced), ½ pound diced mozzarella, ¼ cup grated parmesan, and ½ cup coarsely diced sundried tomatoes. Serve sprinkled with chopped fresh basil.

Wild Mushrooms and Bacon – Use 2 cups sautéed shiitake and baby portobello mushrooms, ½ pound diced crumbled bacon, and ½ pound diced camembert or brie. Top with fresh avocados and lots of coarsely chopped tarragon.

If you run out of ideas for frittata fillings, there are thousands of recipes for frittatas online. Have a looksee.

PALEO WRAPS

These egg wraps can be used like tortillas or crepes. You can fill them with any combination of delicious stuff and healthy stuff, and either roll them into cylinders and cut them, sushi-style or fold them into burritos.

Egg wraps can be served at breakfast, brunch, lunch or dinner, depending on the filling. If you can fill a sandwich with it, you can fill a wrap with it. And they travel well, so you can give them to the kids to eat in the car on the way to school, or include them in a lunchbox.

For each wrap:
1 egg
1 tablespoon cream
A pinch of salt and pepper
Oil for brushing the pan
Parchment or waxed paper

Whisk together the egg, cream and salt and pepper. Heat a non-stick 9- to 10-inch sauté pan over medium heat. Rub with a paper towel or brush the bottom of the pan with enough oil to lightly coat. Pour the egg evenly into the pan. It should sizzle and set almost immediately, making a round egg crepe. Within 20 seconds or so, the bottom of the wrap will be lightly browned and the top surface will appear cooked. Slide out onto a sheet or parchment or waxed paper, top with another sheet of parchment or waxed paper and make more wraps.

To reheat, microwave for 20 to 30 seconds.

Stuff for the wraps:

Tuna or Chicken Salad Wraps – Serve at room temperature.

Sliced ham and cheese – Serve at room temperature, perhaps spread with a little mustard before rolling, or reheat to melt the cheese.

Hamburger/Cheeseburger Rollups – Leftover cooked hamburger or ground beef or turkey, with shredded or sliced cheese, and ketchup or whatever else you like. Microwave on high for 20-30 seconds.

Sliced Roast Beef and Avocado Wrap – Add some chopped tomatoes and serve at room temperature.

Smoked Salmon and Cream Cheese – Add some chopped dill and serve at room temperature.

Asparagus and Swiss – Spread with a little Dijon mustard, if you want, roll up cooked asparagus and Swiss cheese and microwave on high for 20 to 30 seconds to melt the cheese.

Breakfast Sausage or Bacon – Just wrap and serve.

Meats

We recommend that you choose free-ranging or grass-produced meats over feedlot meats wherever possible. The nutritional characteristics of these meats are healthier because of their fat and omega-3 fat content.

A GREAT ROAST BEEF, PLAIN OR RUBBED

Makes 6-8 servings

Prepare the roast plain, with just salt and pepper on the outside or use the Universal Rub (recipe follows) for a more complex flavor. The two best roasts are eye of the rib, prime rib roasts (bone still in) or New York strip roasts. Rib roasts are more tender; strip roasts are firmer and slightly more flavorful.

3 to 4 lbs boneless rib roast or New York strip roast
1/3 cup olive oil
Salt and fresh ground black pepper

Heat the oven to 450°F.

Rub oil all over the surface of the meat, then sprinkle generously with salt and pepper and massage in.

Place the roast, fat-side up, in a roasting pan and cook at 450°F for 30 minutes, then reduce the heat to 350°F and continue to roast for 1 hour to 1½ hours or until the meat thermometer reads 130°F for medium rare – a little longer for medium a little shorter for rare.

When done, carefully transfer the roast to a carving board and allow it to rest for 20 to 30 minutes so the juices can settle back into the meat, then carve.

UNIVERSAL RUB

Makes about 2 cups

This complexly flavored, slightly smoky flavored rub is great on beef, lamb, pork, chicken, and the richer, firm-fleshed fish like salmon and halibut; thus the name universal. Massage it into the meat or fish you are cooking, with some oil or melted butter.

1 cup sweet paprika
1/3 cup smoked paprika
1/3 cup mild chili powder
1½ tablespoons onion powder
1½ tablespoons garlic powder
2 tablespoons ground cumin
1 tablespoon crushed dried rosemary
1 tablespoon crushed dried thyme
1 tablespoon crushed dried marjoram
1 tablespoon freshly ground salt
2 teaspoons freshly ground black pepper

Combine all the ingredients and mix until thoroughly blended. Store in an airtight jar at room temperature for up to 6 months.

ROAST PORK LOIN WITH FRESH HERBS

Makes 4 to 6 servings

A 2½-pound boneless pork loin roast, well trimmed
4 teaspoons finely chopped fresh rosemary
2 teaspoons finely chopped fresh thyme
¼ cup olive oil
Salt and freshly ground black pepper

Heat the oven to 400°F.

Rub the roast all over with olive oil and then massage in the herbs and a generous amount of salt and pepper. Place fat side down in a foil-lined roasting pan. Roast for 30 minutes. Turn roast fat side up. Roast until thermometer inserted into center of pork registers 145°F, about 15 to 20 minutes longer. Remove from oven; let stand 15 minutes so the juices can settle back into the roast, then carve.

Rubbed Pork Roast – Massage about 1/3 cup of Universal Rub into the roast along with the fresh herbs and salt and pepper.

GRILLED OR SAUTÉED BURGERS

Makes 4 burgers

The best burgers are made with ground sirloin that has been seasoned with salt and pepper and then gently formed into patties. Don't overwork the meat when shaping the burgers; gently form it into patties without too much pressure. You can use beef, lamb, bison, buffalo, or even turkey to make these burgers.

1½ pounds ground sirloin
Salt and freshly ground black pepper

Sprinkle the meat with salt and pepper then divide into quarters. Gentle shape each into a patty, without squashing the meat. Obviously, the thicker the patty, the longer it will take to cook. Grill or sauté, then add toppings and garnishes to your liking.

Grilled Burgers – Heat the grill to medium hot. Lightly oil the grill and then lightly oil the burgers. Grill to the desired degree of doneness, for medium rare it will take about 4 minutes on each side, for medium, about 6 minutes.

Sautéed Burgers – Heat a heavy-bottomed pan over medium-high heat. Add the burgers; it's best if they don't touch, so you might want to cook them in two batches. After about a minute, reduce the heat to medium and continue cooking until the burger is deeply browned, then reduce the heat to medium low, flip and cook to the desired degree of doneness. Medium rare burgers will take about 5 minutes in total, medium burgers 7 or 8 minutes.

Some Topping Suggestions:

Have fun with toppings, and remember, there really isn't any reason for a bun. Burgers are just as good, even better, when eaten off a fork rather than your fingers!

- Bacon, avocado and Monterey jack cheese
- Guacamole, cheddar cheese and diced fresh cherry tomatoes
- Goat cheese and watercress

- Swiss cheese, sautéed mushrooms and sour cream
- Red Leister cheese and a fried egg with very thinly sliced jalapeños
- Blue cheese and Sundried Tomato Pesto (see recipe previously)
- Cooked spinach and brie
- Pizza burger for the kids – topped with mozzarella and tomato sauce
- Hot wing burgers – top with the spicy orange meat of boned buffalo wings and ranch or blue cheese dressing
- Outrageous burgers – topped with a slice of duck liver paté and caramelized onions
- Korean burgers – topped with sliced fresh beefsteak tomatoes and kimchi

And, of course, don't forget the lettuce, tomato, onion and pickles. *Do* forget the bun, though.

MARINATED FLANK OR SKIRT STEAK

Makes 6 servings

This marinade adds a mahogany color and a complex Madeira flavor with bursts of garlic and ginger to the flank steak. A few slices of this steak will enliven any family meal or a company dinner. In warm weather, leftovers can be refrigerated and served cold in sandwiches later in the week. Pork tenderloin takes well to this Madeira marinade and is cooked in exactly the same manner.

¼ cup Madeira
¼ cup light soy sauce
2 shallots, peeled
A ½-inch chunk fresh gingerroot
3 garlic cloves, peeled
Juice of ½ lemon
½ teaspoon coarsely ground black pepper
1½ to 2 pounds flank or skirt steak, trimmed

In a food processor, combine the Madeira, soy sauce, shallots, ginger, garlic, lemon juice and pepper and process, pulsing frequently, until all are finely chopped. Pour into a shallow glass dish large enough to hold the flank steak in a single layer.

Place the flank steak in the dish and rub it all over with the marinade. Marinate in the refrigerator overnight for 24 hours, turning occasionally and rubbing each time so the marinade evenly coats the meat. The longer the steak marinates, the more deeply the marinade will penetrate.

Heat the broiler.

Lift the steak over the dish and scrape off the marinade. Pat dry. Place on an aluminum foil-lined roasting pan and slide under the broiler. Broil until medium rare, about 4 minutes on each side. To test for doneness, make a small slit in the meat with the tip of a sharp paring knife. It should be very pink, but not red.

Transfer the steak to a cutting board and allow to rest for 5 minutes before carving.

Carve into thin slices on the bias — across the grain. (Carving the meat this way will make it more tender.)

ROASTED MARINATED LEG OF LAMB FOR A PARTY

Makes about 10 to 12 servings

This is a grand roast for large parties or buffets, with a special cooking process that gives it a richly colored surface. The lamb is marinated to give it additional flavor and to tenderize it in a mixture of oil and soy sauce flavored with lemon, garlic, onions and herbs. A honey glaze flavored with anise is brushed onto the lamb, and then it is roasted to produce a succulent medium-rare interior and a dark, sweet, fragrant crust.

Special note: This recipe requires 2 days of marinating and considerable attention during cooking.

Half a lemon
1 medium-sized onion, peeled and quartered
2 shallots, peeled
4 large garlic cloves, peeled
2 bay leaves, crumbled
1 tablespoon dried rosemary
½ cup olive oil
1 cup soy sauce
½ cup honey
1 tablespoon anise seeds
1 teaspoon freshly ground black pepper
One 6- to 7-pound leg of lamb, trimmed of excess fat and pelvic
    bone removed (ask the butcher to do this for you)

In a food processor, combine the lemon, onion, shallots, garlic, bay leaves and rosemary, and pulse until everything is coarsely chopped. Do not over-process. Pour the oil and soy sauce into a non-aluminum pan or baking dish large enough to hold the lamb leg, add the chopped vegetables, and mix together.

Slip the lamb into the marinade, turning it until it is well coated, then scatter some of the vegetables over the top. Cover and refrigerate for 2 days, turning several times each day to ensure that the leg marinates evenly. Remove from the refrigerator 3 to 4 hours before cooking to allow the lamb to come to room temperature.

Heat the oven to 500°F.

Lift the lamb out of the marinade and scrape the vegetables off the meat. Pat the lamb dry. With a piece of kitchen string, tie the floppy top of the leg (the sirloin end) neatly together and place the lamb on a rack in a large roasting pan.

Strain the marinade and discard the vegetables. Pour 1 cup of the marinade into a bowl and add the honey. Grind the anise seeds finely in a spice mill or electric coffee grinder, or crush well in a mortar. Add the anise and the pepper to the cup of marinade. Beat lightly with a whisk, and pour slowly and evenly over the leg of lamb.

Place the lamb in the center of the oven and roast for 10 minutes. Remove from the oven, turn the lamb over, and quickly baste all round with the marinade from the pan. Slip the lamb back into the oven, reduce the heat to 450° F and roast for 10 minutes. Turn and baste again, then reduce the heat to 400°F and roast for 10 minutes. Turn and baste. Return the lamb to the oven, reduce the heat to 350°F and roast for 10 minutes. Turn and baste again (the basting liquid will have thickened considerably by now), return to the oven, and reduce the heat to 300 °F. Roast until done, turning and basting every 10 minutes. The total cooking time for medium rare meat will be about 12 minutes per pound; for medium, about 14 minutes per pound.

If you do not have an instant-read thermometer, use these minute-per-pound figures to determine when the roast is done. If you do have an instantly registering thermometer, about 10 to 15 minutes before you estimate the roast will be done, insert it into the thickest part of the leg without touching the bone. For medium rare, it should register 130 to 135°F when the lamb is done; for medium, 150 °F.

At this point in the roasting, the internal temperature of the lamb will rise about 1 degree every 1-1½minutes, so in order for the temperature of the roast to increase by 10 degrees it will take 15 minutes.

By the time the lamb is done, the kitchen will be perfumed with its fragrance. Remove the lamb from the oven, lift out of the roasting pan and place on a cutting board, where it should rest for 15 to 30 minutes so the juices can settle back into the meat.

Just before carving, remove the string. Slice and serve.

Posted blog: **Bacon-The New Meat Candy**

"I had rather be shut up in a very modest cottage with my books, my family and a few old friends, dining on simple bacon... than to occupy the most splendid post which any human power can give." Thomas Jefferson

Go ahead; eat like Jefferson–eat 2 or 3 or even 4 slices of bacon with your eggs if you want. Just cut out the toast.

There was a recent spate of articles about the dangers of eating processed meats and how they increase your risk of having a heart attack or getting Type 2 diabetes. They were all based on a press release from the Harvard School of Public Health. The press release, although generally good, is typical public health sensationalism regarding processed meats.

The main problem with the cited studies was that they did not adjust for other dietary habits or socioeconomic status. What that means is that the increased risk for disease probably relates to the generally less healthy diets and lifestyles than to the effects of processed meats. And most of the studies did not distinguish between one type of processed meat and another.

The problem with these sorts of studies is that most people who eat a lot of fast-food-burgers and hot dogs also do a lot of other stuff that's bad for them compared with people who are most likely to sit down to a steak and potato dinner with the family.

Government publication per the "the plate" US Dietary Guidelines and touted by the First Lady, recommends "eating less" red and processed meat. This is based on the completely fallacious belief that eating red meat raises the cholesterol level in our blood and thereby increasing the risk of coronary heart disease, stroke, and diabetes mellitus. This is nonsense; there are forty years of evidence that it is nonsense. (See Addendum for sources)

Let's look clearly and honestly at the nitrites and nitrates which are found in bacon and our belief that they cause serious health problems, especially cancers. In fact, the study that originally connected nitrates with cancer risk has long since been discredited. (See Addendum for sources) There have been major reviews of scientific literature that found no link between nitrates or nitrites and human cancers, or even evidence to suggest that these compounds may be carcinogenic. Recent research suggests that nitrates and nitrites may not only be harmless, they may actually be beneficial, especially for immunity and heart health.

So let's talk about bacon. Put it on your burgers, crumble it in your salads, eat it with your eggs, toss it with your broccoli or Brussels sprouts or spinach, wrap chicken and roasts in it, add it to your pizzas. Bacon really is the candy of the 21st century; delicious, healthy, and an excellent aspect of eating right and *Living in Wellness*.

Whether you're a traditionalist, a perfectionist, or simply seek convenience, you can cook perfect bacon:

The Traditionalist uses the frying pan. Whether it's because of the sizzle or the smell, bacon to them is not bacon unless it's fried in a frying pan on a burner on top of the stove. Maybe they like cooking their eggs in the rendered fat. The bottom line: to the traditionalist, bacon's got to be fried.

How it's done: Lay strips of bacon on the bottom of a cold cast iron frying pan. Don't overlap the strips but cover the entire pan bottom. Cook one side of the strips then turn them over and cook the other side. Remove the bacon strips with tongs and drain on paper towels.

Positives and negatives: There is the undeniable pleasure of sizzle and smell and then there's the bonus of bacon fat for frying the eggs! The uninitiated, however, may end up overcooking or even undercooking the bacon. Still, practice makes for perfection.

The Perfectionist aims for a perfectly flat, crisp product— no curling or twisting. They want it magazine perfect with a restaurant taste.

How it's done: This bacon is cooked in the oven on a broiler tray or the like—something that catches the bacon grease. The method requires that you watch the progress of the cooking as it's happening because 10 to 15 minutes is all it takes.

Positives and negatives: Although less messy and not as prone to spattering as the stove top method, you could end up with charred strips in just moments. However, you do need that right pan for the job.

The Convenience Cook wants it all to happen now. This is a quick, easy method to get your bacon.

How it's done: On a layer of three or more paper towels on a microwave safe plate, lay your uncooked bacon strips and cover with a couple more layers of paper towels. Nuke for 4 to 6 minutes in the microwave.

Positives and negatives: The towels soak up the bacon grease but you could also wind up with a mess in the microwave. The big advantage is that anyone can do this.

All that said, you are now ready to experiment. Try this:

Chocolate Bacon Bars – Melt some bitter chocolate in a double boiler and dip 2" strips of crisply cooked bacon in the chocolate. Serve warm or refrigerate.

Chicken

Chicken being another animal food, we recommend you choose from free-ranging and/or organically grown chickens.

WHOLE ROASTED LEMON CHICKEN

Makes 4 to 6 servings

This is your basic, every-day and even good-enough-for-company roasted chicken: healthy, happy, luscious and easy to prepare. It can also be the source for the chicken used in chicken salads, frittatas, soups, and for any recipe calling for "leftover" chicken. Because dark meat is no longer our enemy, enjoy this more flavorful part of the bird with a new gusto! And the skin too!

A 3-pound chicken
½ cup melted butter
1 small lemon, cut into 8 or 10 pieces
Salt and freshly ground black pepper

Heat oven to 375°F.

Rub the chicken all over with half the melted butter and salt and pepper. Stuff the cavity with the lemons (they will steam and flavor the chicken from the inside). Tuck the wings under the bird (no need to truss the legs).

Place in a foil-lined (for easy cleanup) roasting pan and roast, uncovered 30 minutes. Brush generously with some of the remaining butter. Roast uncovered about 45 minutes longer, brushing once or twice times with the remaining butter.

Testing for doneness: Insert an instantly registering thermometer into the thickest part of the thigh without touching the bone; it should register 160 to 165 degrees.

When done, transfer to a carving board and allow the chicken to rest for 20 to 30 minutes so the juices can settle back into the meat before carving.

For a Rubbed Roasted Chicken – Rub the skin of the bird with Universal Rub, along with the salt and pepper, before roasting.

THAI CHICKEN SALAD

Makes 4 servings

This salad is full of flavor and texture; it can brighten up a scorching-hot day or a dull, rainy summer day. It is at once sweet, hot and sour; soft and crisp, moist and crunchy. For a different taste, substitute a poached or grilled duck breast for the chicken.

Fish sauce, a thin, brown, salty and fishy liquid, is as essential to Southeast Asian cooking as soy sauce is to Japanese and Chinese cooking. Thai fish sauce, called nam pla, and Vietnamese fish sauce, called nuoc nam, are the two most commonly available in the United States, and can be found in supermarkets, specialty stores, and Asian groceries.

2 whole boneless, skinless chicken breasts (about 1 pound total weight), each cut in half lengthwise
2 celery ribs, julienned into 1-inch-long match sticks
1 large cucumber, peeled, seeded, and julienned into 1-inch-long matchsticks
1 small red onion, peeled, cut in half lengthwise, and thinly sliced
A 1½-inch-long chunk of fresh gingerroot, peeled and finely chopped
1 bunch cilantro, very coarsely chopped
2 garlic cloves, peeled and finely chopped
½ small jalapeno pepper, seeded and julienned into 2-inch-long matchsticks
2 tablespoons fish sauce (see note above)
Juice of 4 limes

Fill a medium-sized sauté pan half-full with water. Place over a burner set on high and bring to a boil. Add the chicken, reduce the heat, and simmer for 3 minutes. Turn off the heat and allow the chicken to finish cooking as the water cools, about 20 minutes.

When chicken is cool, either tear into shreds with a fork or cut into thin strips. Toss the chicken with the remaining ingredients.

Serve at room temperature or slightly chilled, but not refrigerator cold, which would harden the proteins in the chicken and make it tough.

Desserts

It seems blasphemous to the cookbook gods not to have any desserts in a cookbook. With a serving of fruit per day as our guideline, and a decided disinterest in stuff that is made with sugars or wheat, desserts become mostly fruit. How we combine the fruits, how we accent them, and whether we accompany them with cheese or nuts or chocolate, or even bacon (yes, crumbled bacon makes almost any fruit better!), is what makes them fun and exciting.

So desserts fall into these areas: fruits, fruit salads and roasted fruit. A few of the latter are included here to point you toward becoming a Paleo-fruit gourmet.

Better yet, it's okay not to have dessert at all. Listen to your body. You should be full after eating a meal of protein, fats, and vegetables. Try to eat what is seasonally appropriate for where you live. The only reason many fruits are available year-round is due to the invention of the airplane. So lower your carbon footprint by avoiding buying blueberries in December in Chicago.

Dr. Kaskel's Little Dessert Secret – Every day after lunch I sit back in my office chair and mindfully eat--and thoroughly enjoy--an 8-gram piece of Dove dark chocolate. My friend Carl Jerome, who wrote the recipes in this book, says a small chunk of Mast Brothers chocolate (available online), Vahlrona or Scharffenberger (available in most supermarkets) is even better! Regardless, eat it mindfully (see Mindful Eating, above).

PAPAYA AND RASPBERRY SALAD

Serves 6

Colorful, textured and fragrant.

1 medium-size, ripe papaya; halved, seeded, peeled and cut into
bite-size chunks
½ pint fresh raspberries
6 to 8 ounces pomegranate seeds
Orange flower water

Gently toss the fruit together then sprinkle with orange flower water.
Serve, or refrigerate until needed.

CANTELOUPE AND BLUEBERRY SALAD

Serves 6

Sweet, tart and refreshing

½ medium-size ripe cantaloupe, peeled, seeded and cut into bite-
    size chunks
1 pint fresh blueberries
½ cup full fat plain Greek yogurt

Toss the cantaloupe and blueberries. Divide onto serving plates and
top with a dollop of yogurt.

STRAWBERRIES WITH PISTACHIOS

Serves 6

1 quart fresh strawberries, hulled and halved or quartered into
    large, bite-size pieces
¾ cup shelled raw pistachios, very coarsely chopped
Grated zest of 1 orange
Juice of ½ lemon
2 Tablespoons extra virgin pistachio oil (optional)
½ cup cold heavy cream, whipped until soft peaks form, optional

Gently toss together the strawberries, pistachios, lemon zest, lemon juice and oil, if using, and serve with or without the whipped cream.

FRESH PEARS AND BRIE

Serves 6

4 large ripe Comice pears, peeled, cored and cut into large dice
4 ounces brie cheese (refrigerator cold), cut into dice slightly smaller
    than the pears
½ cup pine nuts
2 Tablespoons extra virgin pine nut oil, optional

Gently toss everything together and serve, or refrigerate until needed.

Variation – Substitute crumbled blue cheese for the brie, replace the pine nuts with coarsely chopped raw walnuts, and use walnut oil instead of pine nut oil.

BLACKBERRIES AND CHOCOLATE

Serves 6

3½ pints blackberries
1 cup ground bitter chocolate
8 ounces Devon clotted cream or mascarpone cheese, or crème
   fraîche

Gently toss the berries with the chocolate. Divide onto serving plates and top with a dollop of the creamy stuff of your choice.

ROASTED PEARS

Serves 6

4 Tablespoons unsalted butter
6 unpeeled ripe Bosc or Barlett pears, quartered, stemmed
 and cored
Juice of 1 large lemon
1 Tablespoon very finely chopped fresh tarragon
1 cup fresh whole-fat sour cream or crème fraîche

Heat the oven to 425°F. Generously butter a large rimmed baking sheet. Toss the pears and with the lemon juice. Transfer pears, cut-side down, to the buttered baking sheet. Roast 20 minutes. Turn pears, placing other cut-side down. Roast 20 minutes. Turn pears, skin-side down. Roast until pears test just tender, about another 5 to10 minutes.

Divide onto serving plates, sprinkle with a little tarragon and top with dollop of sour cream or crème fraîche.

ROASTED SPICED PEACHES

Makes 6 servings

> 6 tablespoons butter, melted
> 6 firm-ripe peaches, halved and pitted
> 1/4 teaspoon each ground cinnamon, ground coriander and ground
>   cardamom
> 1 large juice lemon

Heat oven to 350°F. Brush half the butter over the bottom and sides of a round glass or ceramic baking dish large enough to hold all the peaches upright. Place peach halves, skin-side up, in dish.

Mix the spices into the remaining butter with a whisk. Fill the center of each peach with half the spice butter. Brush the tops of the peaches with any remaining melted butter. Bake 25 to 30 minutes or until peaches are just tender.

Serve warm or at room temperature, drizzled with pan juices and sprinkled with a few drops of fresh lemon juice.

Variation: Use nectarines instead of peaches.

ADDENDUM

More of Dr. Kaskel's Blogs

Posted blog: *The Illusion of Health and Diets*

You know how when you buy a new car, or are in the process of buying a new car; all of sudden, you see that same car everywhere? That type of car has always been around you, you just haven't noticed it, but now, since you're aware, they're everywhere!

This morning I went to my favorite diner for breakfast. Well, I guess today I lost my sensitization to the people I see daily in my practice for weight loss strategies and started really paying attention to my surroundings. There are really a lot of overweight people out there; some so grossly overweight that I honestly couldn't believe that they haven't succumbed yet. I just couldn't help thinking about why they are the way they are. In my practice I talk to them. They may be genetically predisposed to weight, or others may have an eating disorder, but I firmly believe that both are controllable. And, if it's controllable for them, imagine those of us who don't have issues like they have, what we can do to drop those extra pounds.

I asked my server at the diner if they were putting anything special into the foods that they were serving that would cause everyone to be so heavy. He looked at me and laughed and said, "They're not like you -- you didn't order the bread or potatoes". That's exactly it!

Let's not even talk about potatoes here, let's just focus on bread. Now, I'm not going to go into a long dissertation about bread; it will be short, but if you want the long explanation, it's out there.

Bread: It's a grain. Whole wheat, multi, oat, rye...;it doesn't matter what kind it is, where you buy it, or how you consume it; it's going to have the same physiological effect on everyone's body. The effect is that, once digested, it all turns into sugar. FACT: Sugar turns into FAT in your body. The biochemical mechanism for this is very simple, and it's all about your body trying to rid itself of sugar. It does this by releasing insulin to get it out of your blood stream. Why? Because sugar doesn't belong there! Left there for too long a time it can cause disease. Our bodies are very efficient in ridding themselves of the equivalent of nuclear waste, dumping it in our bellies and behinds (not to mention on our internal organs)? Again, another physiological FACT.

Let's review: Grain = sugar = insulin release = fat storage.

There. In just one line I've written the only and best diet information needed on earth. You can now throw out all of those diet books you've read.

Back to the illusion of health and diets. So, you go into a decent restaurant and they label their menu offerings as "heart healthy" which makes you think that these foods are good for you and if they're good for you, they should not cause you to gain weight! I'm right, am I not? Case in point: What is every breakfast menu comprised of? Of course eggs and bacon (but you're told to stay away from that), so the bulk of the menu items are pancakes, cereals, waffles, crepes, scrambled eggs with hash browns, toast...you get it. So, if all of these offerings are turning into sugar in our bodies and turning into fat, why do we eat them?

Here's my answer. Arrogance!

As American citizens, we are arrogant! I use arrogant to mean we actually think that we know what is good for everyone in a nutritional context. Let's not forget that we are just animals. Sorry! Animals have a limited choice of foods that they are able to consume in order to afford health and weight management. There are no obese animals in nature, except humans and those animals that are fed a human Western diet. As humans, we are meant to eat animals and vegetables, that's it. Throw into the mix all the foods you find either at the grocery store or at most restaurants and do you really think we're able to assimilate those foods that nature didn't intend us to consume?

Again, let's review: any food that is not animal or vegetable = ill health = obesity

Now, we really want to believe that if this stuff we're eating were bad for us, of course someone would have told us not to eat it, right? No! Where does the food money that you spend go to in this country? Is it the meat industry and vegetable industry? No. Is it the processed foods and companies that are producing everything else that you buy that isn't meat and vegetables? Yes! And how do they get you to believe that what you shouldn't be eating and is making you sick and fat is?

They have you reading it in magazines. It's called advertising and marketing. They all do a fabulous job of keeping us sick and fat.

And there's your local "healthy grocery store." They are the worst! I push my cart around these stores like everyone else. You don't have to look at labels when food is on these "healthy store" shelves, because it's implied that it's "healthy"! More arrogance! They are marketing to you the illusion of health because of the name of their store. So, let's look at what is actually in these stores. Let's see. There's a bakery section . . . that's all wheat and flour products (fat). There's the store pizza section (all wheat/grain crust = fat). There's the dairy section (more sugar = fat). Do you see that yet? You're spending more money for products that you think are healthier for you, but you're really just buying and eating the same crap you could get at a gas station mini-mart!

So what are you supposed to do? Here's my answer: Think about yourself and your family and their health and weight. The illusion of a healthy breakfast consists of orange juice, toast and cereal (like Kashi® whole grains and Special K®). All sugar, sugar and more sugar. Lunch is comprised of whole wheat bread, peanut butter and jelly and Gatorade. Sugar, sugar and more sugar. Same thing with dinner: whole wheat pasta, potatoes and Vitamin water. Sugar, sugar and more sugar. There you have it. You are making yourself fat all day eating what you have been brainwashed into thinking is healthy, because you bought it all at a fancy grocery or are eating it at a fancy restaurant.

Do any of these places really care about your health and weight? Or do they just want your money? Hmmmm.

In at least a couple of key respects, we're not much different from cows. It is, for us and for cattle, easier and cheaper if we are raised in an unhealthy way. It is really difficult and expensive to raise healthy cattle. This is why we have meat from unhealthy cattle sold us. Meat from healthy cattle costs more but is good for us. Not only is it good for us, it will actually make us healthier than our prevalent diet, which is laden with unhealthy carbs and sugars.

Again: The press has demonized beef and dairy claiming it is unhealthy. They are wrong.

If I could get on my podium right now and debunk five major myths we have been fed by often well-meaning and well-intentioned but grossly uninformed food writers, this is what I'd say:

Myth: Eating Beef And Dairy Is Unhealthy.

WRONG. Beef and dairy from grass-fed cattle cared for without antibiotics and hormones are healthy products. They have low levels of Omega-6 fatty acids and higher levels of Omega-3 fatty acids. This is also true about pasture-raised lamb and pork and all "red meats."

However, conventionally raised beef and dairy are in fact unhealthy because of what they are fed. They are not meant to eat GMO corn, nor get pumped full of antibiotics and growth hormones. Eating meat and dairy from these animals is unhealthy. We shouldn't be feeding genetically altered corn to animals so they will fatten-up quickly in a way that is harmful to us as their end users.

So look for and buy grass-fed, pasture-raised meat and eat it as often as you like.

Myth: Raising Cattle Is Bad For The Earth And A Poor Use Of Land.

WRONG. A sustainably run ranch is good for all. Cows eat grass and then return nutrients to the soil, which refreshes and replenishes the land. It is environmentally friendly, and a good use of the often rocky and hilly land that would not be appropriate for crops.

Unfriendly to the environment are conventionally tended acres of dusted, sprayed and chemically fertilized croplands.

Myth: Raising Cattle Is Not Humane.

WRONG. There is a humane way to raise cattle: allowing them to roam pastures, grass-feeding themselves, allowing them to grow naturally. More expensive, yes. But the alternative is unhealthy animals and unhealthy protein being sold in our markets.

We need to stop raising cattle in feed lots and tight confines and forcing them to eat unnatural foods. This unnatural diet combined with terrible living conditions leads to enormous levels of disease, thus the need for antibiotics.

It's time to choose the right and humane option here.

Myth: Red Meat Is Bad For Our Hearts.

WRONG. Red meat is actually good for your heart, if the animals from which it comes are raised naturally.

This myth was introduced in the 1950s when we mistakenly began to correlate high cholesterol, saturated fat and heart disease. It has been propagated falsely for 60 years. Since it began in 1948, the Framingham Heart Study, the largest and longest nutritional study in history, has told us this is FALSE, yet we continue to believe it.

If you feed cattle what they are intended to eat, this correlation disappears.

Myth: Plants Can Provide All Our Nutritional Needs.

WRONG. Our bodies are designed to eat animal protein. These proteins are complete with all essential amino acids and high in Omega-3 fatty acids. Plant based omega 3s require our bodies to convert them to useful fuel which is very inefficient. Grass-fed beef is also high in Vitamin D, which is difficult to get from plants.

Can people live successfully as vegetarians? Yes, if they jump through enough hoops, assuming they know which hoops to jump through. The point of *Living in Wellness* isn't to be in a battle with our basic nutritional needs.

Living in Wellness supports eating grass-fed, naturally raised, free ranging cattle. If you are like most of us, you won't have ready access to a grocery that carries healthy red meats and certainly not the variety of animals and meats you would want in cooking for a family. U.S. Wellness is an online source for healthy beef, lamb, poultry, bison, pork, rabbit, etc. Have a look at their web site. Or search online for ever-increasing numbers of ranchers in Illinois, Wisconsin and Missouri who produce healthy cattle and healthy meats and meat products.

In the end, we're not a lot different from cows. We both need to eat right to be healthy.

Interview with Dr. Uffe Ravnskov

Friday October 23rd at 9:00 AM CST

This interview was recorded after my radio show ended. The National Lipid Association would not approve this interview for the "Lipid Luminations" radio show that they sponsored on ReachMD.

Dr. Ravnskov is a Danish independent researcher specializing in cholesterol. He is author of The Cholesterol Myth, *one of the most widely read and respected books on cholesterol and health. He is an independent researcher who has published more than 100 articles and letters in international scientific journals exposing the fallacy that high cholesterol and saturated fats are unhealthy. He is the author of several books on the subject.*

DR. LARRY KASKEL (LK): *"The great tragedy of science is the slaying of a beautiful hypothesis by an ugly fact."*

That was said by Thomas Huxley.

On the homepage of THINCS, The International Network of Cholesterol Skeptics, it reads:

"For decades enormous human and financial resources have been wasted on the cholesterol campaign. More promising research areas have been neglected, producers and manufacturers of animal foods all over the world have suffered economically, and millions of healthy people have been frightened and badgered into eating a tedious and flavorless diet, and into taking potentially dangerous drugs for the rest of their lives. As the scientific evidence and support of the cholesterol campaign is nonexistent, we consider it important to stop it as soon as possible."

Our guest today is Dr. Uffe Ravnskov. Dr. Ravnskov has spent the better half of his career trying to debunk one of the greatest medical myths of all time; the cholesterol myth: That cholesterol is evil and that a diet high in fat is the cause of heart disease.

139

In today's show hopefully we will learn something about the case that things are not always as they appear and that conventional wisdom is often wrong.

I would like to start with some definitions. You have said in your writings that the cholesterol campaign is one of the greatest mistakes in medical science. What did you mean by that?

DR. UFFE RAVNSKOV (UR): What I mean is, cholesterol is considered one of the most important molecules in our body. Cholesterol is the main constituent in our cells. You cannot build a cell without cholesterol. We use it for producing many important molecules. For instance, by changing its structure a little, we are able to convert cholesterol to estrogen, testosterone, cortisol, and vitamin D. Cholesterol is of vital importance for the brain. We cannot think without cholesterol. It is used by the brain cells and the nerve fibers as building materials. In fact, more than half of the brain's dry substance is composed of cholesterol. It is so important that all cells are able to produce it themselves. We produce 4 to 5 times more cholesterol than we eat. If we eat too little, our production goes up. If we eat too much cholesterol, it goes down. That is the reason why it is so difficult to lower it by dietary means.

LK: How did you first get interested in this topic and even looking at the use of statins and the fact that we exaggerate their benefits, that they have been abused, overused, and misused for so many years?

UR: I have followed the literature in this area meticulously for more than 20 years. In 1992 I published a review of all of the cholesterol-lowering trials that had been published at that time, a total of 22, in the *British Medical Journal*. It was a few years before the statins were introduced. When I took all of the results together I found that cholesterol was not able to lower heart mortality. In fact, if you put all the results together, total mortality was higher in the treatment groups. Those who took notice argued that cholesterol was not lowered enough. Already at that time many other studies had shown that high cholesterol was not the cause of heart disease. I just might mention that several post mortem studies have shown that people with low cholesterol are just as atherosclerotic as people with high cholesterol.

LK: Right. I think it is well known that half of the people that come in with a heart attack have low cholesterol and half of them have high cholesterol.

UR: Recently, a large American study was published. The authors had measured cholesterol in 137,000 patients admitted to hospital because of a heart attack and found that it was lower than normal. Another research group confirmed their findings and concluded that their cholesterol had to be lowered even more. They did that, but three years later they found that there were twice as many who had died among the half whose cholesterol had been lowered the most, compared with the other.

LK: So in 1992 you looked at 22 trials that really showed no decrease in mortality. Now we are in 2009 and there have been many more trials done. Do you have any conclusions as to the benefits of statins now, in 2009?

UR: There is a small benefit, but the benefit is only for people who already have had a heart attack and it is trivial. For instance, if you are 60, your chance of being alive during the next five years is about 85%. But, if you take a statin every day you can improve your chance to about 87%. These figures are true only for people who have already had a heart attack. If you are healthy and your only so-called "problem" is high cholesterol, a statin agent cannot prolong your life, it can only lower your risk of getting a non-fatal heart attack and, again, the effect is trivial. But at the same time, you are exposed to the many side effects from such treatment. We all know that a non-fatal heart attack is not that serious. It often heals without serious consequences.

LK: I'm sorry. I think most people that are taking this pill are taking it to extend their life and not have a fatal heart attack.

UR: Yeah, yeah, but again, this is only true if you already have had a heart attack. It is not true for healthy people with normal or high cholesterol and it is not true for women either. The problem is that the side effects are underrated because they do not come immediately. It might take several months before they appear and at that time neither the patient nor the doctor think that they are caused by the drug, instead they blame increasing age. People are told that side effects are rare, that they are mild; but what is happening is that the experts are belittling them. For instance, the most common side effect is weak and painful muscles. These episodes occur in less than 1% according to the trial directors, but independent researchers have recorded that at least 25% complain of muscle problems. Another side effect is erectile dysfunction. This is also said to occur in less than 1%. However there is a study paid by Pfizer and they found that 20% of the male patients become more or less impotent after a few months' treatment. If you go to the homepage of Lipitor, Pfizer's statin drug, there is not a word about impotency, but of course as you know they have another billion-dollar drug to solve that problem called Viagra

LK: Right, exactly.

UR: There are other side effects that are not known by most doctors because they are not mentioned, but many, many cases of mental disturbances have been reported, as well as back pain, depression, nightmares, and even memory loss. However for some curious reason, these side effects have never been reported to the general population or to doctors. The most serious side effect is cancer. We have known for many years that low cholesterol is a risk factor for cancer. If you treat mice and rats with cholesterol lowering drugs, they get cancer also. Except for two early trials, what happened in all of the other trials that have been published after these two, the trial directors have ignored to report the number of skin cancers. It is very discouraging because if we think that statins or cholesterol-lowering agents can induce cancer, the first type of cancer we should see is skin cancer, because it is so easy to see when it comes. I mean,

LK: Can we get back to the actual theory that because the whole world believes it and the research seems to support it, that high fat diets cause heart disease. How can so many people be wrong, or, as the expression goes, "How can ten million Frenchmen be wrong?"

UR: That is a good question because there is absolutely no support whatsoever to that idea. There are at least 30 cohort studies that have shown that patients with heart disease have not eaten more saturated fat than healthy people. Even more interesting is that at least 8 studies have shown that stroke patients have eaten less saturated fat than healthy people; no study has found the opposite. Now if you go to the previous WHO [World Health Organization] recommendations, the main argument is that saturated fat raises cholesterol. This is not true either and you can read about that in my new book. Even if it were true, high cholesterol is not a disease. Recently, a few weeks ago, the WHO published a new paper about which diet to recommend. Now the experts have changed their minds and I quote, I have that report in front of me, "The available evidence from cohort and randomized controlled trials is unsatisfactory and unreliable to make judgment about and substantiate the effects of dietary fat on risk of coronary heart disease." But, in the conclusion, they have not changed their recommendations. They still recommend less than 10 cal percent of saturated fat.

LK: How can we fight this and deprogram or un-brainwash our society to the fact that cholesterol and saturated fat is not evil and that there is no such thing as good and bad cholesterol?

UR: That is a good question, but I can't give you an answer because this is what I and my group have tried almost in vain for 20 years. Myself, I have published numerous scientific papers and also a number of books in seven different languages, written for lay people, and very little has happened. Perhaps this program and radio show will reach them. I hope so.

LK: It seems that there is [a] subtle shift now going on that the concept of inflammation initiating and continuing the disease is being accepted, but they are still not letting go of LDL and now LDL being oxidized as the new enemy. I personally have always thought of LDL as just being a poor innocent bystander caught up in the accident, but not the initiating cause.

UR: Yes, I agree with you. I think you are right. Many or most researchers are inclined to mention factors associated with LDL as a risk factor and consider them as the cause. I used to say that firemen, are often seen where houses burn, but they are not the cause of the fire. Now they have focused on oxidized cholesterol, but I think this is a way to keep the cholesterol myth going. There is no evidence that oxidized cholesterol is the cause either.

LK: So, in your opinion Dr. Ravnskov, what is the initiating event that causes the damage of the endothelium thus setting up the chronic inflammatory process?

UR: We all agree that, as you say, inflammation is present in the artery wall before atherosclerosis appears, but in my view there is no doubt that atherosclerosis is an infectious disease. More than 50 different bacteria and a lot of viruses have been identified in atherosclerotic arteries, but not a single one in normal arteries. If you ask patients with an acute heart attack or stroke, about one third of them will recall that they had an infection just before they became sick. Another argument is that periodontal infections are a strong risk factor for heart disease. Recently, Italian researchers have reported that after they treated the infected teeth, there was significant improvement of the arteries in these people. In my view, the inflammation in the arterial walls is not the very cause, it is secondary to infection. How else do you explain that treatment with anti-inflammatory drugs increase the risk of heart disease? The inflammation is caused by the microorganisms and it is a necessary step for the healing process, it is not the cause.

LK: So, is there any way to, in the living person, isolate what is growing in their plaque and if you treat them with antivirals or antibiotics, can you make a difference? Can it penetrate into plaque?

UR: There are several trials where researchers have tried to prevent heart disease with antibiotics, but as you see more than 50 different bacteria and many viruses have been isolated. It is very unlikely that you can do anything this way and they have not succeeded either, save for a few times.

LK: What about just vaccinating better?

UR: Yes, there are a few trials where people have vaccinated patients and these have indeed shown positive results. In fact, much better than statin treatment.

LK: Right. I have seen studies where if you immunize against the flu you can get a 6% absolute risk reduction and I have never seen anything like that in a statin trial. Doctor, you recently published an article in the *Annals of Clinical and Laboratory Science* entitled, "Vulnerable Plaque Formation from Obstruction of Vasa Vasorum by Homocystinealated and Oxidized Lipoprotein Aggregates Complexed with Microbial Remnants and Auto Antibodies." Can you dumb this down a little for my audience? Translate that into English and discuss what it means.

UR: I will try. First, I published the paper together with Kilmer McCully. Kilmer is the guy who discovered that high homocysteine was more important than high cholesterol. He was kicked out of Harvard and lost his funding when he published his first paper about that. He was unable to get a new position for 1½ years. However, as you know the role of homocysteine has been acknowledged by now by most researches and fortunately Kilmer has been acknowledged, as well. Our idea is based on the fact that the lipoproteins; HDL, LDL, and VLDL partake in immune system by binding and inactivating bacteria and virus and their toxic products. This has been verified again and again by a dozen research groups starting more than 50 years ago. Obviously, very few know about it. You cannot find a word about it from the current experts. The problem with this system is that in case of prolonged or severe infections, the microorganisms aggregate together with the lipoproteins. The aggregates become larger if the patient also has high homocysteine levels because homocysteine changes the LDL molecules in a way so they attract each other. So, all together these processes produce large molecule aggregates and they have great difficulty passing the capillary. In particular those that supply the artery walls, the vasa vasorum. What we think is that the vasa vasorum in the arteries become occluded by these complexes and the artery wall becomes ischemic; then the microorganisms escape into the wall and cause inflammation. In the worst scenario, we think that a vulnerable plaque is created and as you probably know, we have known for many years that blocking off an artery almost always occurs where a vulnerable plaque has burst and emptied its content into the artery. What we claim is that the vulnerable plaque is a microscopic boil. Morphologically, they look like boils and, just like boils in the skin, they are warmer than the surrounding tissue. Many of the symptoms in patients with acute myocardial infarctions are the same as with infectious diseases. They get a slight fever, leukocytosis, sweating, and even chills. In severe cases it has been shown that about 20% of the patients have bacteremia or sepsis.

LK: What do you see as the most powerful intervention available today, in 2009, that we can use to decrease one's risk of dying from cardiovascular disease?

UR: Well, I do not know for sure, but there are several risk factors for heart disease and they are still there. Our hypothesis is that stress, for instance, raises cortisol and cortisol predisposes us for infection. Smoking predisposes for all kinds of infections and diabetes does the same. How to prevent this? Well, stop smoking. Try not to be mentally stressed. Exercise is probably a good idea. The problem is that many people are unable to exercise because of the muscle side effects from statin treatments.

LK: Stay away from human beings that you might get an infection from?

UR: Yes, yes, of course. You should not actually exaggerate the role of infections. Most of us get infected now and then all through life. But if we could find something that strengthens our immune system, it is a good idea.

LK: Doctor, do you think that when the statin patents run out there will be a window of opportunity where we can reeducate physicians and populations of the world that the diet-heart hypothesis was just that; a hypothesis and that it was actually wrong?

UR: I do not think that price or patent questions have any influence. Most doctors and lay people all around the world have been brainwashed and they are willing to pay anything, in money and manpower, to save us from the devil cholesterol. I think something radical will happen when people realize that their muscle problems, their bad memory, bad temper, their sexual failure, bad libido or their cancer are caused by the drugs they have been prescribed. I should tell you what has happened in Sweden. A few years ago a general practitioner treated her own obesity with a low-carbohydrate diet with a high content of animal fat. When she gave similar advice to her obese and diabetic patients, she was reported to the National Board of Health and Welfare for malpractice. Fortunately, there were some wise people there and she was acquitted, because her treatment was considered to be in accord with scientific evidence. Many trials have now shown that the best way to treat type II diabetes is a low-carbohydrate, high-fat diet. Several books have been published here in Sweden by authors who have achieved a dramatic improvement of their health by a similar diet. This has gained general attention due to a number of reasons. These authors, and also some of us, have debated with the official experts. The effect has been that the intake of butter, cream, and animal fat are increasing in Sweden after many years of decline. A recent study showed that a majority of Swedes think that the best way of losing weight is by a low carbohydrate fat-rich diet. What I mean by telling that is that the [medical and food] industry never changes their mind, but when lay people discover the bad effects from statin treatment and the benefit of fat food on their own bodies, I am sure something will happen.

LK: That leads me to my last question. I am a lipidologist in the United States and I live in a very litigious society. I worry about getting sued and I get letters from insurance companies even telling me that I am not writing enough statins if I am not. How [am] I, as a lipidologist who has been indoctrinated by the cholesterol campaign, supposed to go out and apostatize to the world when I do not even believe the theory, how do I avoid becoming a fringe physician and be able to explain this intelligently to my patients and teach them the realities of the limitations of statin therapy?

UR: That is a different issue. I assume that even [in] the United States it is the patients who decide whether they should follow the doctor's advice or not. It is not the doctor who demands them to take this or that drug. So, if you tell your patients honestly about the trivial benefits they can achieve by statin treatment and the many side effects, I am confident that no one wants you to prescribe such drugs. What I will warn against is to tell people to stop statin treatment because anyone can die suddenly whether on statin treatment or not and if that happens, you may be accused of malpractice. So, inform the patient instead or you could ask them to read my new books. This is also my advice to those who think that I am crazy.

LK: Can you tell us the name of your new book?

UR: My new books are *Fat and Cholesterol Are Good for You!* and *Ignore the Awkward! How the Cholesterol Myths are Kept Alive.*

LK: I am just curious – before I go – what is your cholesterol level and do you take a statin?

UR: My own cholesterol is almost 300. I am not taking a statin, no, and I am eating eggs and milk and butter and cream.

LK: How young are you?

UR: I am 75.

LK: Excellent. Well, I thank you very much for your time, Dr. Ravnskov.

Recommended Reading:

This is a list of books that Mike and I have read and that go into greater detail on the science and literature behind our dietary guidelines. We owe all these authors our gratitude for waking us up to reality. Thank you all.

All of these books are currently available for purchase online, either in print or electronically.

Wheat Belly by William Davis, M.D.

Good Calories, Bad Calories by Gary Taubes

The Blood Sugar Solution by Mark Hyman

Why We Get Fat by Gary Taubes

The Art and Science of Low Carbohydrate Living by Stephen Phinney and Jeff Volek

The Art and Science of Low Carbohydrate Performance by Stephen Phinney and Jeff Volek

The New Atkins for a New You by Eric Westerman, M.D., Stephen Phinney, M.D.

The Paleo Solution by Robb Wolf

The Primal Blueprint by Mark Sisson

Deadly Harvest by Geoff Bond

Fat and Cholesterol Are Good For You by Uffe Ravnskov, M.D.

Ignore the Awkward by Uffe Ravnskov M.D.

Genocide by William Carlson M.D.

Primal Body, Primal Mind by Nora Gedgaudas

Protein Power by Dan Eades

Cereal Killer by Alan Watson

Eat Fat, Lose Fat by Mary Enig

Fats Are Good for You by Jon Kabara

Is Your Cardiologist Killing You? by Sherry Rogers, M.D.

Sweet Poison by David Gillespie

Life Without Bread by Christian Allan and Wofgang Lutz

Big Fat Lies – Is Your Government Making You Fat? By Hannah Sutter

Cholesterol and Saturated Fat Prevent Heart Disease by David Evans

Low Cholesterol Leads to an Early Death by David Evans

Biographies

Larry Kaskel, M.D. is Medical Director of Northwestern Wellness Center in Libertyville, IL. He attended Rush Medical College and did his Internal Medicine residency at Rush Presbyterian St. Luke's Medical Center in Chicago, finishing in 1991. He is board certified in internal medicine and board certified in clinical lipidology. He has been in private practice since 1991.

Dr. Kaskel is an expert in using Therapeutic Lifestyle Change for his patients and has lectured extensively on this topic, both in the United States and internationally.

He has hosted and recorded more than 300 radio shows on ReachMDXM, a satellite radio channel for medical professionals. Currently, he writes a blog, www.livinginwellness.org, and remains passionate about treating patients with his philosophy of "More Education and Less Medication."

He is married, has two young children, and lives in the northern suburbs of Chicago.

Michael Kaskel is a Registered Nurse practicing nutrition, weight loss and diabetic education for Northwestern Wellness Center in Libertyville, IL. He received his nursing degree from Loyola University in Chicago.

Mike began his nursing career in a hospital setting caring for severely ill patients, but felt his strengths were better utilized with patients in a disease-prevention model than a disease management role.

With his preventative approach towards wellness, he has succeeded in turning around the lives of thousands of patients through education, not medication, without the use of often-recommended "supplements" to offset health issues. He strongly believes that our current health system is rife with misconceptions and blatant mistruths about nutrition that affect all of us in some way. He works daily with patients to educate and move them towards a more healthful way of life.

Made in the USA
Coppell, TX
06 November 2020

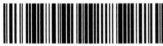